Medical English for Communication

コミュニケーションのための 医学英語

Daniel Velasco, Ph.D.
ダニエル・ヴェラスコ
〔著〕

朝倉書店

Medical English for Communication

1st Edition

ISBN: 978-4-254-30128-1 C3047

Preface — To the Student

This textbook is intended for students who are studying in a medical school, nursing school, or any other program related to medicine. Students who have a basic-to-intermediate understanding of English and who wish to improve their English communication skills within medical settings will benefit from this textbook. It contains fifteen units that give students opportunities to improve their English skills while thinking about, discussing, debating, presenting, and writing about topics and issues related to medicine.

While this textbook focuses on the medical field, it is important to understand that it does not teach medicine or medical procedures. The aim is to improve English communication and understanding through exercises and activities using the four skills: reading, writing, listening, and speaking.

All of the units have the following sections:

- a list of medical terms and expressions in English and Japanese (漢字 and ひらがな, and カタカナ), as well as vocabulary exercises;
- a grammar review and related exercises;
- a reading about a topic related to medicine, as well as reading exercises;
- a writing activity;
- a listening activity (with a video);
- speaking strategies (summary); and
- a final unit assignment.

The **Speaking Strategies** sections are only summaries, but the entire sections and activities are available from your instructor. He or she may not include them in your lessons, so feel free to request the complete section, and practice the speaking strategies on your own.

There are many reasons why doctors, nurses, and other medical professionals need to understand and speak English:

- There are actually two types of medical English to consider: English spoken between medical professionals and English spoken to or by patients (laypeople, or non-medical professionals).
- As the world globalizes, more people are moving to foreign countries. The number of foreigners in Japan is expected to quadruple by 2040!

- English is the "common language" in medicine (medical terminology) .
- International conferences often use English as the language of delivery.
- Important and widely read medical journals are entirely or partially written in English. If you want to publish a paper in a medical journal, you will most likely need to submit your paper in English.
- Many medical students have a desire to help people in countries that lack doctors and nurses. Humanitarian groups, such as Doctors Without Borders (Médecins Sans Frontières) , require volunteers to speak English.
- Besides moving to a foreign country to work, many people decide to live in a foreign country for other reasons (e.g., marriage, political instability) . Many countries use English as their main or secondary language.

Within this textbook, there will also be opportunities to learn and practice:

- non-verbal communication, which is helpful when trying to interpret patients' body language;
- pronunciation, intonation, and word stress, which will help convey sympathy, compassion, and important points to your patients; and
- awareness of other cultures, including differing views on medicine and medical practices.

Lastly, a big part of learning medical English is memorizing prefixes, suffixes, and root words of medical terms. Although this textbook covers a lot of medical English terms and phrases (there are 40 in each unit) , it does not cover many prefixes, suffixes, and root words. Therefore, it is recommended that the lessons in this book are supplemented with a highly concentrated study of prefixes, suffixes, and root words. Your instructor may recommend a medical terminology book or prepare supplementary activities that will support your learning.

As you go through the book, sometimes only the term "doctor" or "nurse" is used, but please remember that this book can be used for other medical professionals, including physical therapists, pharmacists, technicians, specialists, psychiatrists, caregivers, and even dentists!

Lastly, as you begin your studies in the medical field, always remember

> *"to rise above the routines of the daily ward round and to see in every patient an opportunity ... to serve mankind in the best tradition of medical excellence."*
>
> —Harvey (1973)

Help Along the Way

Throughout the textbook, you will hear from real medical and nursing students, doctors, nurses, and academic lecturers, as well as real patients.

Also, this is Fushigi-chan! She will be your guide to help you think about and discuss various topics in the medical field.

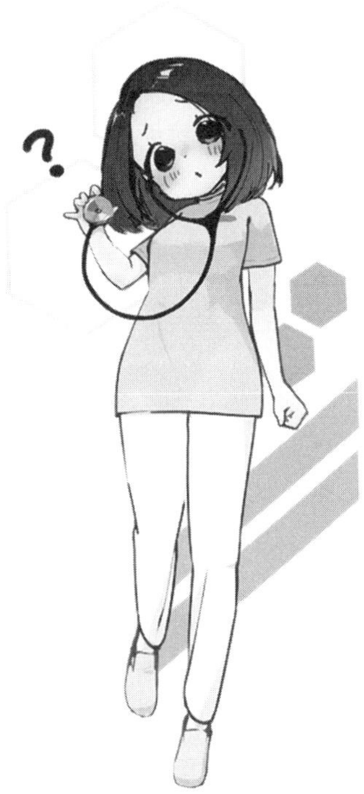

「初めまして！　フシギです．フシギちゃんと呼んでください．
私は人体の神秘にとても魅了され，医療分野に関連する様々なトピックを楽しく学んでいます．各章の新しいトピックについて私と一緒に考えてみませんか？
皆さんも一緒に考え，クラスメートと議論してください . . . もちろん英語で．よろしくね．」

It's nice to meet you! I'm Fushigi. Please call me Fushigi-chan. I'm a medical student who is fascinated with the mysteries of the human body. I enjoy learning about various topics related to the medical field. Join me as I talk about new topics in each chapter. I hope that you can think about these topics with me and discuss them with your classmates...in English, of course.

Contents

Page

UNIT 1

Why Get into Medicine?

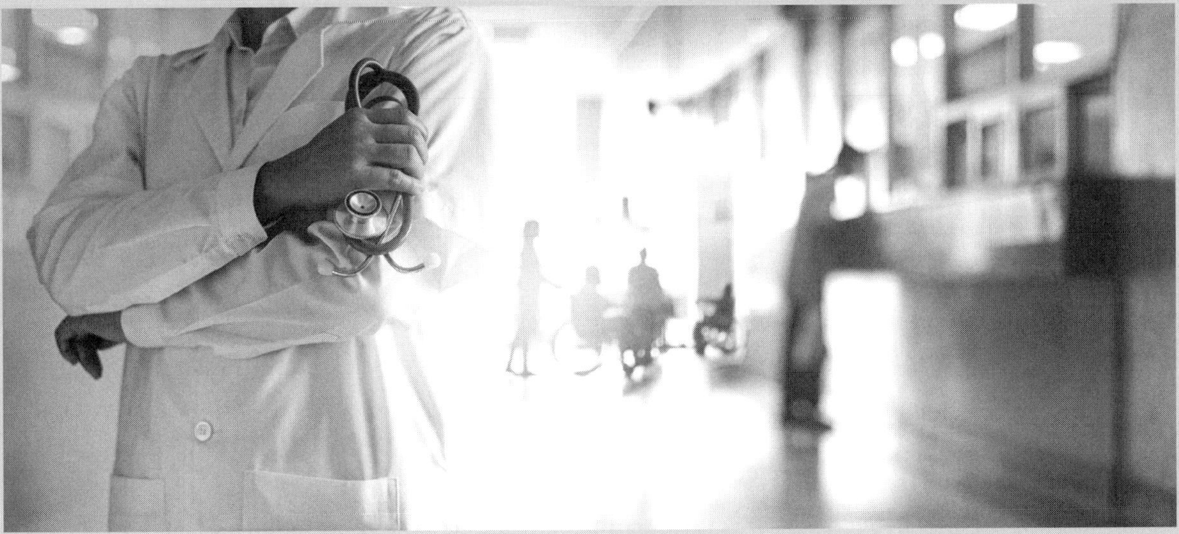

Medical Terms

1. head	頭（あたま）
2. forehead	額（ひたい）
3. eyebrow	眉（まゆ）
4. eyelid	瞼（まぶた）
5. eyelash	まつ毛（まつげ）
6. eye	目（め）
7. nose	鼻（はな）
8. lips	唇（くちびる）
9. mouth	口（くち）
10. chin	下顎（したあご）
11. ear	耳（みみ）
12. jaw	顎（あご）
13. neck	首（くび）
14. shoulder	肩（かた）
15. armpit	脇（わき）
16. arm	腕（うで）
17. elbow	肘（ひじ）
18. wrist	手首（てくび）
19. hand	手（て）
20. finger	指（ゆび）
21. thumb	親指（おやゆび）
22. nail	爪（つめ）
23. chest	胸（むね）
24. nipple	乳首（ちくび）
25. breast	乳房（ちぶさ）
26. abdomen	腹部（ふくぶ）
27. belly	お腹（おなか）
28. navel	へそ
29. shoulders	肩（かた）
30. back	背（せ）
31. hips	腰（こし）
32. buttocks	臀部（でんぶ）
33. thigh	大腿（だいたい）
34. leg	脚（あし）
35. knee	膝（ひざ）
36. calf	ふくらはぎ
37. shin	すね
38. foot	足（あし）
39. heel	踵（かかと）
40. toe	足の指（あしのゆび）

Medical Terms: Practice

Match the medical terms (1-10) to their Japanese translations (a-j).

1) thigh	•	•	a. へそ
2) eyebrow	•	•	b. 臀部（でんぶ）
3) back	•	•	c. 肩（かた）
4) heel	•	•	d. 背（せ）
5) eyelid	•	•	e. 顎（あご）
6) shoulders	•	•	f. 大腿（だいたい）
7) armpit	•	•	g. 脇（わき）
8) navel	•	•	h. 眉（まゆ）
9) jaw	•	•	i. 踵（かかと）
10) buttocks	•	•	j. 瞼（まぶた）

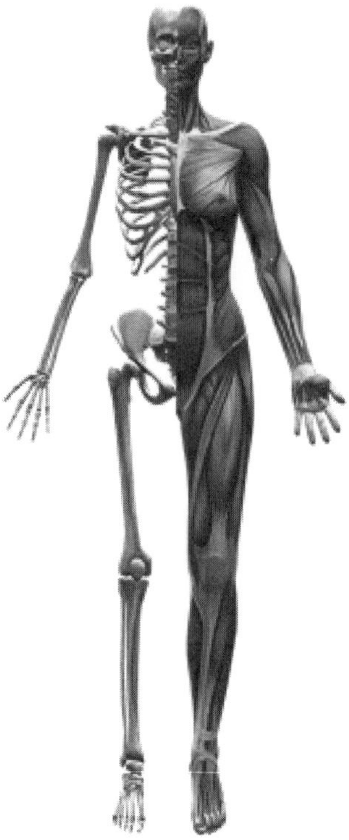

From the list above, how many body parts can you identify? Label the image above with as many parts as you can.

Grammar Review: The verb *be*

The verb *be* has three present forms:

I **am** a medical student. (I'*m* a medical student.)

It **is** a children's hospital. (It'*s* a children's hospital.)

We **are** studying to be nurses. (We'*re* studying to be nurses.)

Not is added to make the sentence negative:

I **am not** good at biology. (I'*m not* good at biology.)

She **is not** from Fukuoka. (She *isn't* from Fukuoka.)

They **are not** in the same school. (They *aren't* in the same school.)

As you can see in the examples above, there are two forms. The full form (e.g., *I am*) is used in formal situations, like writing an essay, and the contracted form (e.g., *I'm*) is used in informal situations, such as conversations and casual writing.

Lastly, you can use *be* with nouns, adjectives, and numbers:

- *be + noun* to talk about jobs and to identify things.
  I **am** a teacher. It **is** a Medical English class.
- *be + adjective* to describe people, places and things.
  The patient **is** sick.
- *be + number* to talk about ages.
  My grandparents **are** both 79 years old.

• Grammar Activity 1

Complete the dialogue with the correct form of the verb *be*. Use *not* for negative sentences.

Student A: It's nice to meet you. My name ___________ Takashi.

Student B: Nice to meet you, Takashi. I'______ Ken. You'______ Japanese, right?

Student A: Yeah. I'______ originally from Tokyo, but I came to Osaka to study medicine. And you?

Student B: Actually, my father _________ Japanese and my mother ________ American. I live in Los Angeles, but came to Japan to study abroad for a year.

Student A: Oh, __________ you in the medical program, too?

Student B: No, I'm studying in another department. My major __________ Japanese literature.

Student A: That sounds interesting! Wait ... it' _____ 3:00. __________ you supposed to be in class right now?

Student B: Oh, thanks for reminding me. It __________ a good thing I'_____ __________ in the medical program. I'd be late for all my classes. Talk to you later, Takashi!

• Grammar Activity 2

Read the sentences and circle the subject pronoun (he, she, it, they, etc.) that refers to the underlined word.

1. My wife and I are sick. **We / They** will go to the hospital today.
2. My mother is a nurse in a big hospital. **It / She** is always late for dinner.
3. When you turn left, you will see the clinic. **It / She** is next to a pharmacy.
4. Risa and Satomi are in the same class. **We / They** are both 21 years old.
5. Dr. Watanabe's lessons are so fun. **They / He** are full of interesting activities.

• Grammar Activity 3

Unscramble the words and phrases to make sentences.

1. the / near / open / clinic / campus / today? / Is / women's

____

2. pediatricians. / Dr. / her / daughter / are / and / Baba / both

____

3. you / late / medical / for / Why / lecture? / are / the

____

4. son / My / in / not / a / heart / becoming / is / interested / surgeon.

____

5. patient / well / surgery. / The / after / not / his / is / doing

____

Reading with Fushigi-chan: Why Medicine?

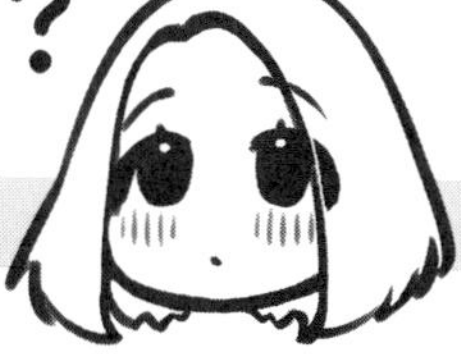

Why do people become doctors and nurses. Medical students have to overcome a lot of difficult obstacles in order to become a doctor or nurse. Four-to-six years of medical school (depending on the country and program) , intense training, internships, and difficult exams are just some of the challenges medical students face. Not to mention the cost of medical school is very expensive. So why do some people choose to go through all these difficulties to become medical professionals?

There are a lot of reasons people decide to get into the medical field. When asked why they decided to study medicine, many medical students would probably answer this question by saying, "I want to help people." Helping others is a great reason to study medicine, and becoming a professional in the medical field is a direct way that they can assist people in a community.

Speaking of community, another reason some people decide to become a medical professional is the status they hold in society. Medical doctors, for example, are trusted members of society, and it is an honorable profession to enter. Doctors have a lot of influence on patients and their loved ones, and earn a lot of respect.

Another thing they earn besides respect is money. Doctors are one of the highest paying professions in the world, so it is natural that many people would choose this career path. Job security and high salaries are what everyone wants in a career, so becoming a medical professional is a good way to secure both.

Lastly, medicine is a fascinating subject. Becoming a doctor means conducting research to learn all about the human body, how it works, and how it sometimes doesn't work. Learning about the body, exams, surgeries, medicines, and the tools and machines that can help people live better and longer lives means that the job will never be boring.

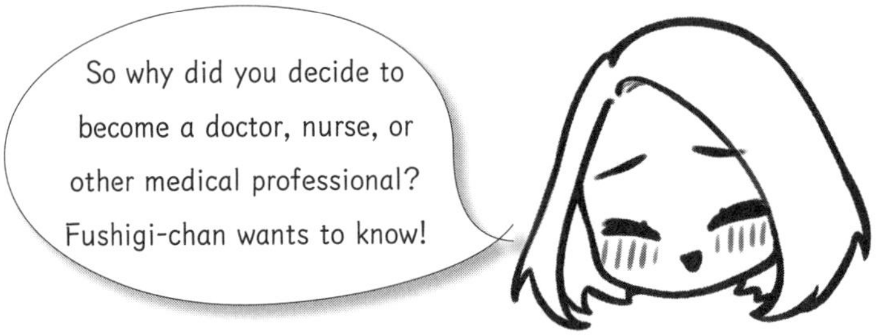

• Reading Activity 1

Circle (T) if the statement is true or (F) if the statement is false.

1. Becoming a medical professional is easy and dull. (T・F)
2. Medical school usually lasts between four to six years. (T・F)
3. Money isn't a factor when some people think about becoming doctors. (T・F)
4. Medical professionals are respected members of society. (T・F)
5. Learning how the body fails is also part of becoming a doctor. (T・F)

• Reading Activity 2

Fill in the blanks with the appropriate words.

1. Another word for something that is challenging that must be overcome in order to achieve a goal is a (n) ________________ .
2. A (n) ________________ is when a student or trainee works in a position, sometimes without getting paid, in order to gain valuable real-world experience.
3. A reason some people decide to become medical professionals is the high status they will hold in ________________ .
4. Doctors are one of the ________________ ________________ jobs in the world.
5. Learning about how the body sometimes doesn't ________________ is also a part of a medical education.

Writing Activity

Write a self-introduction（自己紹介）using the verb ***be***. What is your name? Where are you from? What is your hobby? Who is in your family? Do you have any pets? What's your favorite food? Write 4 or 5 sentences in the box below.

When you're finished, share your introduction with a partner or the class.

Listening Activity

Listen to two students talk about why they decided to become medical professionals. After you listen, answer the questions below. Write in complete sentences.

Speaker 1

1. What is the student's name? What year is she in? What is she studying?

2. What event happened in the student's life that made her decide to study medicine?

3. What is the second reason the student gives for wanting to become a medical professional?

Speaker 2

4. What is the student's name? What year is she in? What is she studying?

5. What reasons does the student give for studying medicine? What skills does she hope to acquire in medical school?

6. Where is the student planning on practicing medicine? What does she want to do after she finishes working as a doctor?

Speaking Activity

What makes a good doctor or nurse?

Think about the qualities or characteristics that make a good doctor, nurse, or other medical professional. Also, think about the qualities or characteristics that make a bad doctor, nurse, or other medical professional. Discuss three good characteristics or habits, as well as three bad characteristics or habits with a partner or small group. After your discussion, work together to complete the lists below. You can also work alone. After you finish, share your responses with the class!

Three characteristics or habits good doctors, nurses, or other medical professionals have:

1. ____________________
2. ____________________
3. ____________________

Three characteristics or habits bad doctors, nurses, or other medical professionals have:

1. ______________________________

2. ______________________________

3. ______________________________

Which qualities, characteristics, and habits were mentioned the most in class?

Discussion Questions

1. Based on the previous activity, what do you believe is the most important quality doctors or nurses should possess? Why? How will you develop this quality?

2. Think about the two speakers in the **Listening** section. Which person's story impressed you the most, and why? Discuss the details you remember, and how they had a positive impact on you.

3. Review the medical terms with a partner or small group. Choose ten words and take turns explaining each word. In other words, teach each other the meanings of the words. Give an example sentence for each word you choose.

Speaking Strategies: General Speaking Skills, Part I

The first step to becoming a good speaker is not the words you use, but the way you use your body. How you sit or stand, where you look (or don't look) , and the way you move your hands are all extremely important when speaking to people. Whether it's one person or a roomful of people, all these parts are important.

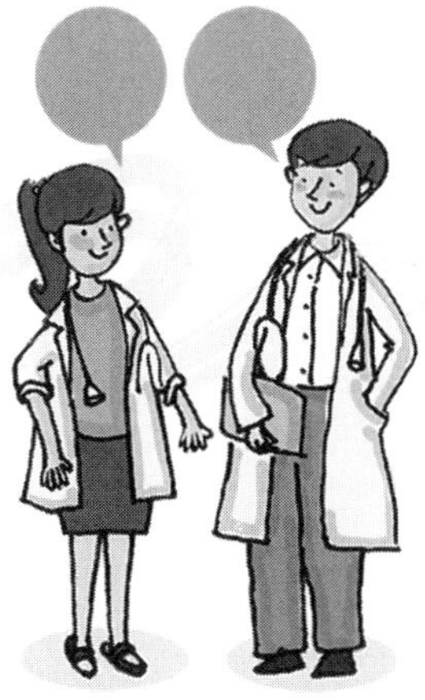

Final Unit Assignment

Topic

Why did you decide to become a doctor, nurse or other medical professional?

Explain why you decided to become a medical professional. Think about the moment you made this decision, and then tell the story. Remember to use details (names, places, dates, etc.) to make your story come to life. Lastly, be sure to use the correct form of the verb *be*, as well as words and phrases you learned in this chapter.

UNIT 2

Working in Hospitals and Clinics

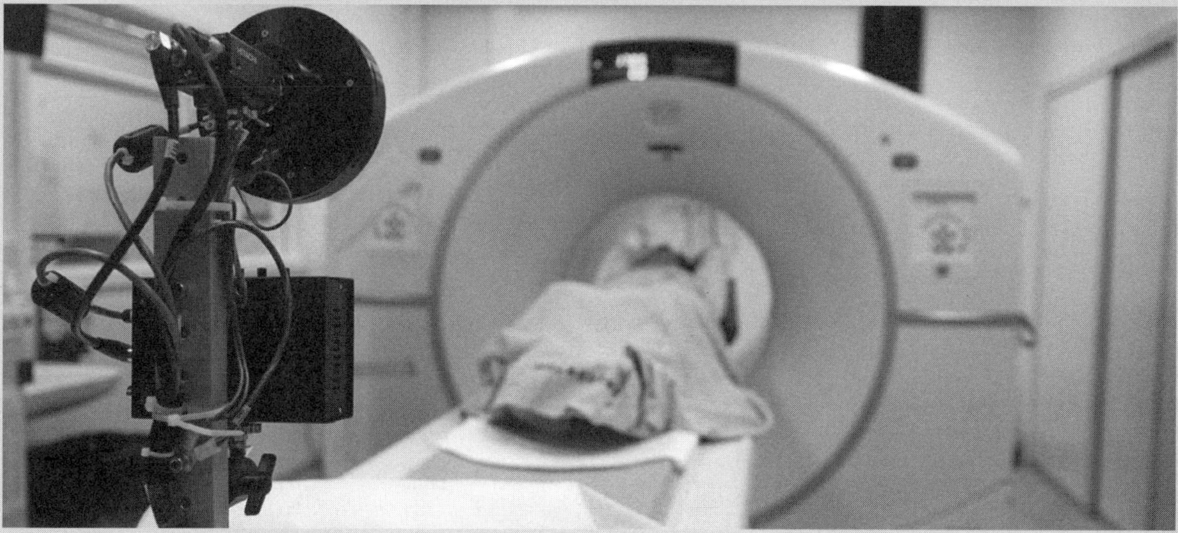

Medical Terms

1. blood vessels	血管 (けっかん)
2. arteries	動脈 (どうみゃく)
3. veins	静脈 (じょうみゃく)
4. capillaries	毛細血管 (もうさいけっかん)
5. aorta	大動脈 (だいどうみゃく)
6. heart	心臓 (しんぞう)
7. left / right atrium	左 / 右 心房(さ / うしんぼう)
8. left / right ventricle	左 / 右 心室(さ / うしんしつ)
9. blood	血液 (けつえき)
10. valve	弁膜 (べんまく)
11. erythrocyte (red blood cell)	赤血球 (せっけっきゅう)
12. leukocyte (white blood cell)	白血球 (はっけっきゅう)
13. brain	脳 (のう)
14. meninges	髄膜 (ずいまく)
15. cerebrum	大脳 (だいのう)
16. cerebellum	小脳 (しょうのう)
17. spinal cord	脊髄 (せきずい)
18. throat	喉 (のど)
19. tongue	舌 (した)
20. gums	歯茎 (はぐき)

21. tooth	歯 (は)
22. trachea	気管 (きかん)
23. larynx	喉頭 (こうとう)
24. tonsils	扁桃腺 (へんとうせん)
25. lung	肺 (はい)
26. diaphragm	横隔膜 (おうかくまく)
27. esophagus (gullet)	食道 (しょくどう)
28. stomach	胃 (い)
29. large intestine	大腸 (だいちょう)
30. small intestine	小腸 (しょうちょう)
31. duodenum	十二指腸 (じゅうにしちょう)
32. nerves	神経 (しんけい)
33. pupil	瞳孔 (どうこう)
34. iris	虹彩 (こうさい)
35. cornea	角膜 (かくまく)
36. spleen	脾臓 (ひぞう)
37. kidneys	腎臓 (じんぞう)
38. pancreas	膵臓 (すいぞう)
39. liver	肝臓 (かんぞう)
40. appendix	虫垂 (ちゅうすい)

Medical Terms: Practice

Match the medical terms (1-10) to their Japanese definitions (a-j).

1) ____capillaries •		• a. first section of the small intestine
2) ____spleen •		• b. area of flesh around the roots of the teeth
3) ____red blood cells •		• c. "food pipe"; an organ through which food passes to the stomach
4) ____esophagus •		• d. a pair of soft tissue located at the back of the throat
5) ____gums •		• e. responsible for controlling the pupil, and gives our eyes color
6) ____duodenum •		• f. cord-like bundle of fibers that send information to the body
7) ____meninges •		• g. connects arteries and veins
8) ____tonsils •		• h. erythrocytes; delivers oxygen to the body through the blood
9) ____nerve •		• i. the three membranes that surround the brain and spinal cord
10) ____iris •		• j. an organ in the abdomen that stores and filters blood, and makes white blood cells

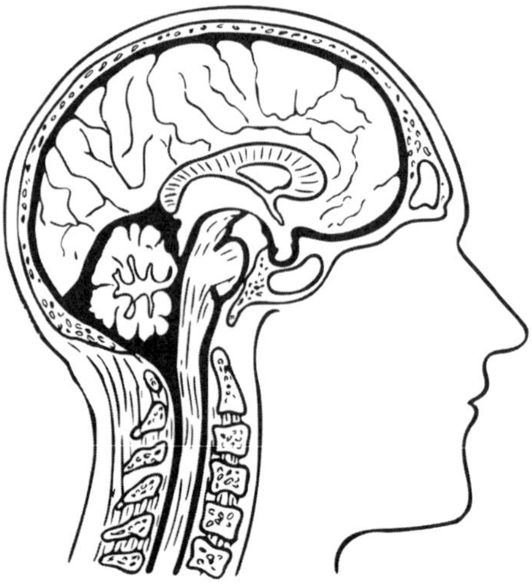

Grammar Review: Nouns and Adjectives

It's important to know the difference between nouns and adjectives.
A **noun** is a word that can be a person, a place, or a thing

I'm a **doctor**.
It's a **hospital**.
This is a **desk**.

Doctor, *hospital*, and *desk* are all nouns.
Nouns can be singular (only one) or plural (more than one) .

Singular nouns	Plural nouns
I'm a **doctor**.	We are **doctors**.
It's a **hospital**.	These are **hospitals**.
This is a **desk**.	These are **desks**.

Adjectives describe or give more information about nouns.

He is a **kind** doctor.
This is an **old** hospital.
These are **wooden** desks.

Kind, *old*, and *wooden* are all adjectives.

Adjectives usually come before nouns, as in "He is a *kind* doctor." Adjectives can also come before the verb *be*, as in "These desks are *wooden*." You can use adjectives to describe the age, color, length of time, shape, and size of people and things.

Also, adjectives have the same form for singular and plural nouns:

Singular	Plural
He is a **kind** doctor.	They are **kind** doctors.
This is an **old** hospital.	These are **old** hospitals.
This is a **wooden** desk.	These are **wooden** desks.

Lastly, adjectives have the same form for singular and plural nouns:

Noun	Adjective
arthritis	arthritic
muscle	muscular
surgery	surgical
meninges	meningeal
cell	cellular

• Grammar Activity 1

Complete the dialogue with the noun or adjective form of the word in parentheses.

Receptionist: Good afternoon, ma'am. Do you need ____________ (help) ?

Patient: Yes, I do. I'm feeling a bit ____________ (fever) .

Receptionist: I'm sorry, could you speak more ____________ (slow) ?

Patient: I think I have a ____________ (fever) . My body is ____________ (ache) and I have a ____________ (sore) throat.

Receptionist: OK. Do you have an ____________ (appointment) ?

Patient: I don't. I tried calling, but no one answered the phone. I only heard this ____________ (annoy) beeping sound.

Receptionist: I'm so sorry. That sound means all our phone lines are ____________ (busy) .

Patient: That's OK. I hope that I can see the doctor soon.

Receptionist: Of course. Please have a seat. The doctor will see you shortly.

• Grammar Activity 2

Complete the noun and adjective chart. If you need help, use a medical dictionary. Write the words in Japanese in the last column.

Noun	Adjective	日本語
1.	atrial	
pericardium	2.	
ventricle	3.	
4.	arterial	
blood	5.	

• Grammar Activity 3

Choose the noun or adjective form of the medical term in parentheses. In some cases, both can be used.

1. Takashi's mother provides (**pediatric / pediatrician**) care. She loves helping children.

2. The patient is experiencing (**muscle / muscular**) pain.

3. Dr. Ogawa is planning to teach us about the (**skeleton / skeletal**) system.

4. Patients call a (**myocardium / myocardial**) infarction a "heart attack."

5. Post-surgery care sometimes involves (**diet / dietary**) restrictions

Reading with Fushigi-chan: Hospitals vs. Clinics

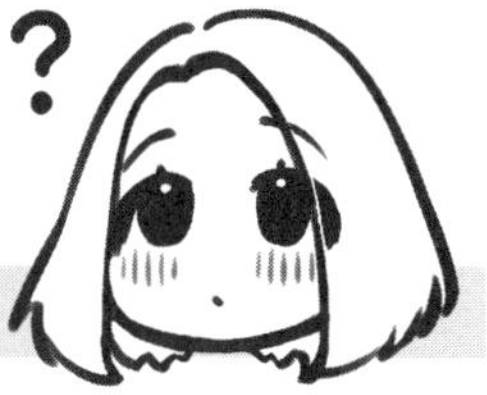

Have you thought about the differences between working in a big hospital and working in a small clinic? If someone is studying to become a doctor, nurse, or other medical professional, they've probably wondered which one would be the best place for them to work.

The obvious difference between a hospital and a clinic is the size. Working in a large hospital would provide many opportunities to work with a variety of specialists. One day, you could work with an x-ray technician, and the next day you could work with a psychiatrist (精神科医, せいしんかい). Every day would bring new chances to learn something new from interesting people who may have different interests and experiences in the medical field.

On the other hand, working in a small clinic means that you will most likely be one of a few doctors or nurses (or maybe the only doctor, if it is your own clinic). While you may not have as many opportunities to meet new professionals with different medical backgrounds every day, you will most likely be working with a small team consisting of receptionists, administrative assistants, nurses, and interns that will surely grow very close over time. This type of environment can make the workplace nurturing and supportive and give a family-like feeling that even patients will experience and enjoy.

Another difference is, of course, the patients. Working in a large hospital means doctors, nurses, and other medical professionals will be extremely busy taking care of many patients. Many patients will leave the hospital after receiving treatment, and new patients will replace them, so it may be difficult to form close connections with them. This is not a negative point, as some people may prefer this to a close-knit workplace. Also, treating a very large group of people with different medical issues will help you learn more about medicine and make you a more confident and competent medical professional.

Location is another area that needs to be considered. Usually, small clinics are located in local communities, so patients are often the same people who will always come to you first for help. The great thing about this is that you really get to know your patients, and may even help multiple generations in the same family (for example, the grandparents, parents, and children) .

There are many other differences that one should think about, including salary, working schedule, commute, and administrative matters (for example, rules, regulations, paperwork, and so on) . Some people may feel restricted working in a small clinic that is located in a rural area, while others may feel lost working in a busy hospital located in the middle of a large urban area.

There are so many obvious differences between hospitals and clinics, but it is important to remember that there are many similarities, as well.

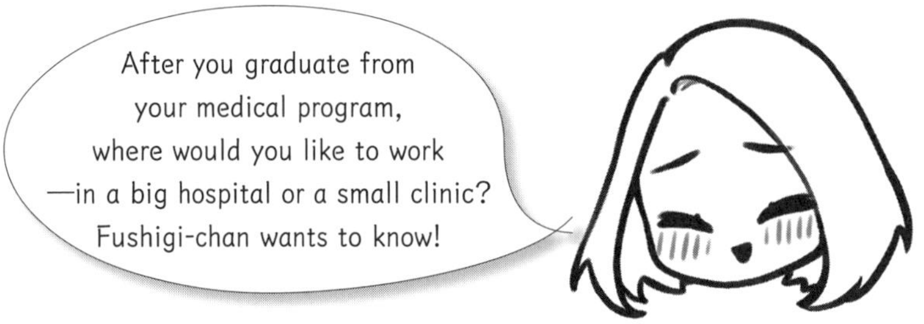

• Reading Activity 1

Finish these sentences about hospitals and clinics, and then explain each point.

1. One of the positive points about working in a hospital is

2. One of the possible negative points about working in a hospital is

3. One of the positive points about working in a small clinic is

4. One of the possible negative points about working in a small clinic is

• Reading Activity 2

Find the adjectives that complete these questions.

1. What are the differences between working in a ____________ hospital and working in a ____________ clinic?

2. Why will many patients leave the hospital after receiving treatment, and ____________ patients will replace them?

3. Why is helping ______________ generations in the same family a good point of working in a clinic?

4. How can working in a clinic create a ________________ and ________________ environment?

5. If you work in a hospital, how can every day bring chances to learn from ____________ people who may have ____________ interests and experiences in the ___________ field?

Writing Activity

After you become a medical professional, where do you think you want to work? You can choose a large hospital or a small clinic, and use the information in the Reading section to help you answer this question. However, you can also choose another healthcare facility—for example, a hospice home（ホスピス）or a mental healthcare facility（メンタルクリニック）. Write 4 or 5 sentences in the box below. Be sure to include adjectives in your sentences.

When you're finished, share your writing with a partner or the class.

Listening Activity

Listen to a doctor talk about the benefits of starting his own clinic. As you are listening, fill in the missing information.

1. When people from overseas come to Japan, some get sick or have ______________, and find themselves dealing with language and ___________ differences in Japanese hospitals and clinics.

2. First, working in a hospital can provide many opportunities to work in various ________________ and ______________. Therefore, hospitals can provide a more ________________ work environment.

3. Second, working ______________ vary between hospitals and clinics. Hospitals are open 24 hours a day, 7 days a week, and there are always ______________ to care for.

4. ______________ shifts are common in hospitals, as is being ________________. Being ______________ means you are ready and available to work when the hospital needs you.

5. There are many other aspects to consider: hospitals are ______________ work environments compared to small clinics; hospitals accept patients with medical ______________ any time, but clinics usually have an ______________ system; and hospitals are usually able to offer higher ______________ than small clinics.

Speaking Activity

Find a partner and ask him or her the questions in **Reading Activity 2**. When you're finished, have your partner ask you the questions. Try to give a different answer or rephrase your partner's answer using different words.

Discussion Questions

1. Describe an average day at a clinic. What do you think a typical day would look like? What kind of problems do you think could happen?

2. Describe an average day at a large hospital. What do you think a typical day would look like? What kind of problems do you think could happen?

3. In pairs, assign roles to you and your partner (patient and staff member). Write a short script like the one at the beginning of the unit, and then act out your script with your partner.

Speaking Strategies: General Speaking Skills, Part II

In the previous unit, we discussed using your body in ways that convey a positive, confident message to your listeners. In this unit, we'll be looking at how to use your voice to further convey confidence, but also to add clearness and emphasis. We will look at two points in this unit: clarity and volume.

Final Unit Assignment

Topic

Difficulties at Work

Conduct research on where you want to work after graduating from medical school (for example, a children's clinic or mental health facility). First, describe some of the job duties. Next, describe some of the difficulties of working in this kind of setting. Be prepared to discuss what you've found to a small group and/or to the class.

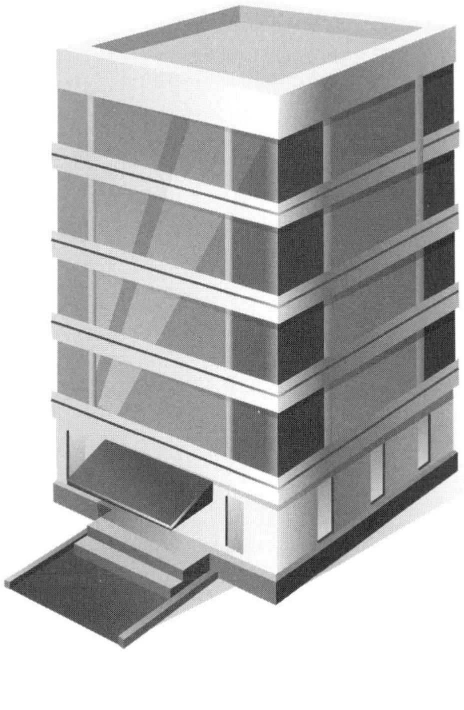

UNIT 3

The Human Body, Part 1

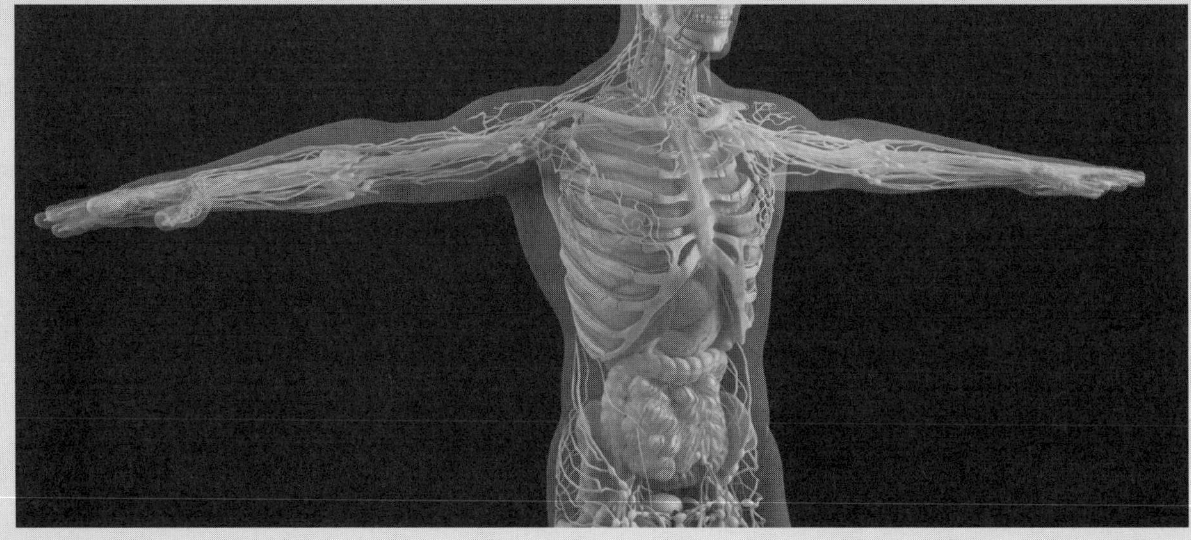

Medical Terms

1. musculoskeletal system	筋骨格系 (きんこっかくけい)
2. circulatory system	循環器系 (じゅんかんきけい)
3. respiratory system	呼吸器系 (こきゅうきけい)
4. lymphatic system	リンパ系 (りんぱけい)
5. nervous system	神経系 (しんけいけい)
6. digestive system	消化器系 (しょうかきけい)
7. urinary system	泌尿器系 (ひにょうきけい)
8. sensory system	感覚器系 (かんかくきけい)
9. biliary system	胆道系 (たんどうけい)
10. female reproductive system	女性生殖器系 (じょせいせいしょくきけい)
11. male reproductive system	男性生殖器系 (だんせいせいしょくきけい)
12. muscle	筋肉 (きんにく)
13. cartilage	軟骨 (なんこつ)
14. ligament	靭帯 (じんたい)
15. tendon	腱 (けん)
16. bones	骨 (ほね)
17. cranium	頭蓋骨 (ずがいこつ)
18. spine	背骨 (せぼね)
19. ribs	肋骨 (ろっこつ)

20. clavicle	鎖骨 (さこつ)
21. scapula	肩甲骨 (けんこうこつ)
22. pelvis	骨盤 (こつばん)
23. femur	大腿骨 (だいたいこつ)
24. patella	膝蓋骨 (しつがいこつ)
25. tibia	脛骨 (けいこつ)
26. fibula	腓骨 (ひこつ)
27. hormones	ホルモン
28. vagina	膣 (ちつ)
29. fallopian tube	卵管 (らんかん)
30. uterus	子宮 (しきゅう)
31. ovary	卵巣 (らんそう)
32. penis	陰茎 (いんけい)
33. testicles	睾丸 (こうがん)
34. scrotum	陰嚢 (いんのう)
35. spermatozoon	精子 (せいし)
36. semen	精液 (せいえき)
37. prostate gland	前立腺 (ぜんりつせん)
38. (urinary) bladder	膀胱 (ぼうこう)
39. urine	尿 (にょう)
40. feces	大便 (だいべん)

Medical Terms: Practice

Circle the words that patients would use to describe these medical terms.

1) patella	a. knee bone	b. kneecap	c. knee joint
2) clavicle	a. collar	b. collarbone	c. scapula
3) mammary	a. breast	b. chest	c. nipple
4) scapula	a. scalpel	b. shoulder	c. shoulder blade
5) urine	a. feces	b. pee	c. urinate
6) spine	a. backbone	b. back	c. spinal
7) femur	a. thighbone	b. tibia	c. fibula
8) cranium	a. bonehead	b. skull	c. skeleton
9) spermatozoon	a. hormone	b. spermatoid	c. sperm
10) feces	a. poo	b. urine	c. anus

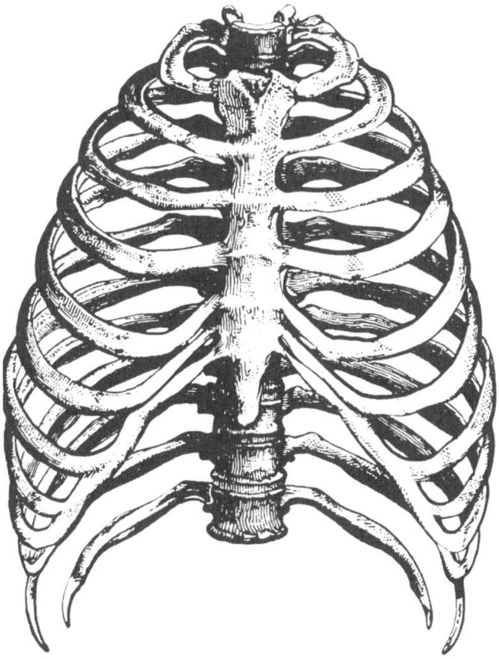

Grammar Review: Simple Present

We use the simple present tense to talk about habits and routines.

I **study** medicine.
She **exercises** after her shift at the hospital.
The chemistry professor **takes** the bus to work.

We use do/does not + verb to say habits and routines we don't do.

I *don't* **learn** medical English from YouTube videos.
He *doesn't* **ride** a bicycle to the hospital.
The students *don't* **watch** medical dramas on TV.

When patients talk about presenting complaints (i.e., problems they are having, and the reason why they are coming to see a doctor) , they can use the simple present to describe something that they are experiencing on a regular basis.

I've **got** a headache.*
I **get** really bad headaches in the evening.
When I **sit** down, my legs **hurt**.

* This tense is considered the Present tense, although it uses the auxiliary verb have. This tense is referred to as the Present Perfect, but the goal is to report an action or event that started in the past (the headache) and is still happening in the present (currently my head still hurts) .

• Grammar Activity 1

Complete the dialogue with the correct words from the box below.

wake	eat	exercise	got	stand	sleep

Student A: I missed my first lesson this morning.

Student B: Really? What time do you usually ___________ up in the morning?

Student A: 5 a.m.

Student B: Wow, that's really early! Why don't you ___________ until 6?

Student A: Because I ___________ every morning to stay healthy. After, I always ___________ a balanced breakfast.

Student B: What was the problem today?

Student A: I've __________ a stomachache and couldn't even get out of bed.

Student B: When you __________ up, does your stomach hurt?

Student A: No, only when I lie down.

Student B: You should go to the school nurse. Maybe he can help.

• Grammar Activity 2

Work with a partner. Ask your partner these questions about their habits and routines, and then write his or her answers below.

My partner's first name: ________________

Question 1: When do you usually get up in the morning?

____

Question 2: Do you eat breakfast every morning?

____

Question 3: How many hours a day do you study?

____

Question 4: What is something you don't do every day?

____

• Grammar Activity 3

Work with a new partner and share the answers from your previous partner in **Grammar Activity 2**. Write down your new partner's information for the same questions.

My new partner's first name: ________________

Question 1: When do you usually get up in the morning?

____

Question 2: Do you eat breakfast every morning?

____

Question 3: How many hours a day do you study?

Question 4: What is something you don't do every day?

Reading with Fushigi-chan: Mysterious Appendix

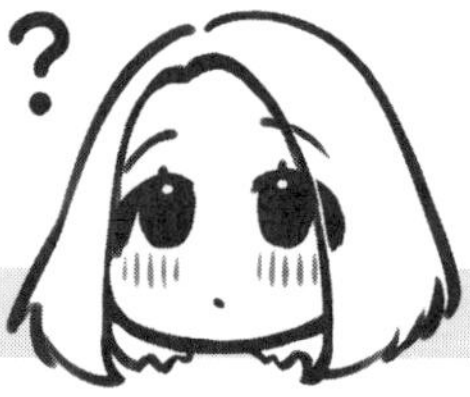

The human body is like a complicated machine, but unlike a machine, which can be disassembled and completely understood, there are many mysteries about the human body that medical professionals and scientists still don't understand.

One of the biggest mysteries of the human body that has puzzled scientists for many years is the organ called the appendix (虫垂, ちゅうすい). The appendix is a thin tube about 10 centimeters long and is located where the large intestine and small intestine meet. So technically it is a part of the gastrointestinal tract, often referred to as the GI tract.

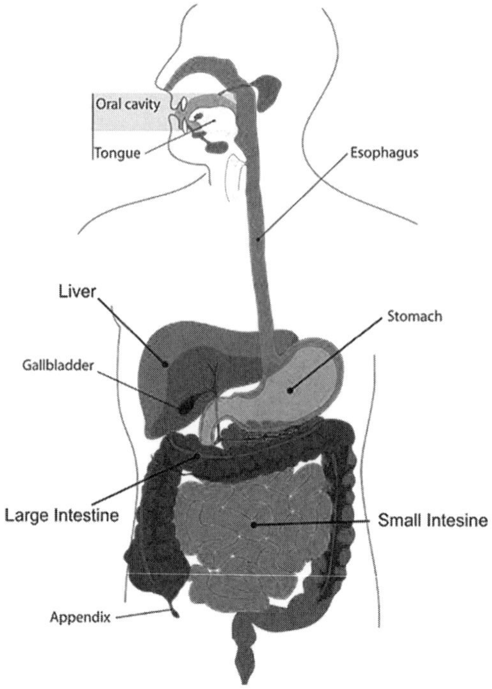

The GI tract helps the body digest food and is made up of two sections. The upper GI tract consists of the esophagus, the stomach, and the duodenum, or the first part of the small intestine. The lower GI tract consists of the rest of the small intestine, and the large intestine, which includes the colon, rectum, and anus. The entire system (including some other important organs, such as the mouth, pancreas, and liver) is called the digestive system.

However—and this is the mysterious part about the appendix—it doesn't seem to serve any function. In other words, although the appendix is part of the gastrointestinal tract, it doesn't actually help the human body digest food.

Why the human body still has an appendix is part of the mystery. Some scientists believe that the appendix used to have a function, but that function disappeared over time through evolution. There are some theories about what the appendix actually does for the human body, including recent research that it functions as a reservoir for intestinal bacteria (Kooij, et al., 2016) , but these are still theories. In other words, the appendix continues to be a mystery.

One thing that the appendix does do for some people is cause problems. Sometimes the appendix becomes inflamed, and people start to feel terrible pain in the lower right side of the stomach or in the navel area. This inflammation is called *appendicitis*. If a person has an appendicitis, this is considered a medical emergency and doctors must remove the appendix as soon as possible. This procedure is called an *appendectomy*. However, because the appendix doesn't play an important role in the body, people can live without it.

The appendix is certainly a great mystery of the human body, but there are many more amazing and unknown things that we still haven't quite figured out.

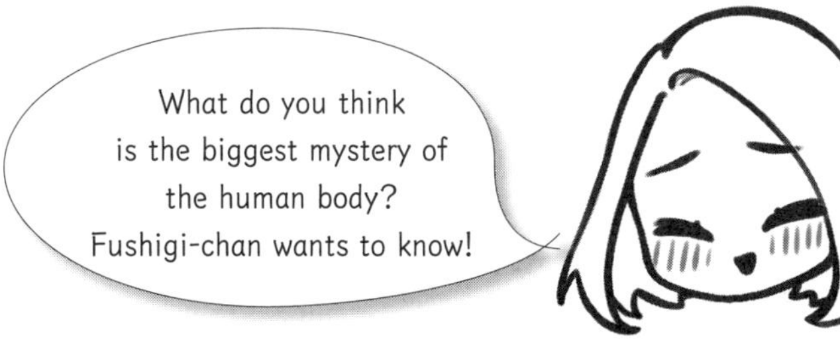

• Reading Activity 1

Circle (T) if the statement is true or (F) if the statement is false.

1. Scientists know the exact function of the appendix. (T・F)
2. The appendix is located at the end of the small intestine. (T・F)
3. According to the reading, some scientists believe that, centuries ago, the appendix had the same function as it does now. (T・F)
4. There are several theories about the function of the appendix. (T・F)
5. The appendix is part of the gastrointestinal (GI) tract. (T・F)

• Reading Activity 2

Match the words and phrases in the box below to their meaning. If you're not sure of the meaning, find the words in the reading section and try to figure out their meaning from the words around them.

puzzled	complicated	referred	disassemble	function

1. ____________________ unable to understand; confused
2. ____________________ to take apart; deconstruct
3. ____________________ consisting of many different parts; intricate
4. ____________________ mention; talk about
5. ____________________ purpose for a specific person or thing

Writing Activity

The appendix is a mysterious organ, isn't it? As the reading states, some scientists believe the appendix used to have an important function but lost its use over time. Write 4 or 5 sentences about what you believe the function of the appendix used to be many years ago. Do you believe it helped with the digestive system or the immune system, or do you believe there was never a function?

When you're finished, share your ideas with a partner or the class.

Listening Activity

Listen to a part of an online lecture on another mystery of the human body. After you listen, read the statements below and circle true or false.

1. For every ten cells, there are ten microbes in the average human body. (T・F)
2. All microbes affect the body in harmful ways. (T・F)
3. There are microbes that help our skin and stomach. (T・F)
4. One to three percent of our body weight is made up of microbes. (T・F)
5. Researchers understand the function of all microbes in the body. (T・F)

Speaking Activity

Different cultures have different beliefs about the human body. Some of these beliefs are based on spirituality (精神性, せいしんせい), superstitions (迷信, めいしん) or false beliefs. As medical professionals, you must be able to explain many things clearly and respectfully while separating fact from fiction.

Think about your own culture or a culture you know very well. What are some beliefs about (or connected to) the human body? The beliefs can be from bedtime stories, myths, fables, popular sayings, or superstitions. For example, a popular saying that is still repeated by many parents in Japan to their children is “If you lie down after eating, you will turn into a cow.” In America, a popular saying that relates to health is “An apple a day keeps the doctor away.”

Discuss two or three more with a partner or small group. Write down what they are, how they are connected to the body, and what are their deeper meanings. You can write notes below while you talk.

- ____
  ____
- ____
  ____
- ____
  ____

Discussion Questions

1. What part of the human body interests you the most? Why?
2. Think about one of the systems of the human body (the nervous system, respiratory system, circulatory system, digestive system, etc.) . Share all the information you know about it. What are some questions you still have about this particular system?
3. After you become a doctor, nurse or other medical professional, what do you think will be one of the most common problems many people will have? Why do you think this problem will be so common?

Speaking Strategies: General Speaking Skills, Part III

Now that you’ve understood the importance of your body when speaking, and hopefully have practiced a lot, it’s time to practice intonation. Intonation is basically how your voice sounds when you’re having a conversation—the tone of your voice rises and falls. This rising and falling tone gives our words meaning and helps our speakers to *feel* what we’re saying.

Final Unit Assignment

Topic

Health Problems

Have you or someone you know had health problems in the past? Of course, we all have been sick or known someone who became sick. The human body is amazing, but it is not a perfect system. Many things happen and people become very sick. However, because the human body is so amazing, people can also overcome their problem and become healthy again.

Talk or write about a health issue in the past that was overcome. You don't have to share private information—for example, you can talk about a sick person from a TV show or movie. Talk about what happened from a medical perspective. What were the symptoms, how did the doctor diagnose the problem, what was the treatment, and how long did it take for the person to heal?

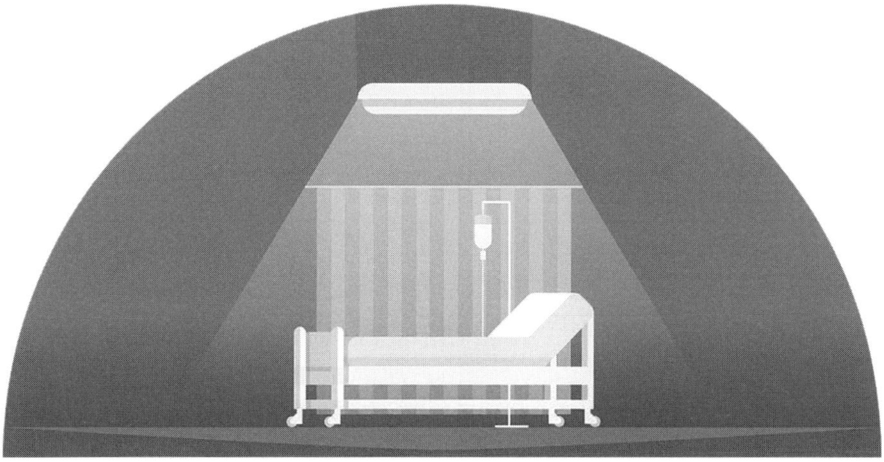

UNIT 4

The Human Body, Part 2

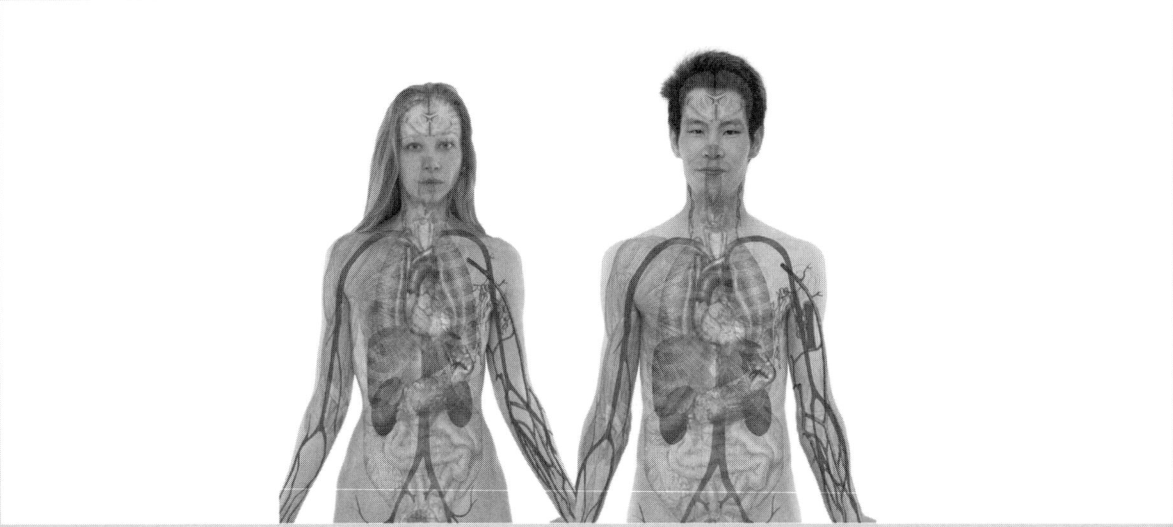

Medical Terms

1. touch	触覚 (しょっかく)
2. taste	味覚 (みかく)
3. sight	視覚 (しかく)
4. hear	聴覚 (ちょうかく)
5. smell	嗅覚 (きゅうかく)
6. breathe	呼吸 (こきゅう)
7. cough	咳 (せき)
8. sneeze	くしゃみ
9. yawn	欠伸 (あくび)
10. chew	噛む (かむ)
11. swallow	飲み込む (のみこむ)
12. digestion	消化 (しょうか)
13. metabolize	代謝 (たいしゃ)
14. belch	げっぷ
15. hiccup	吃逆 (しゃっくり)
16. drool	涎 (よだれ)
17. pass gas	おならをする
18. urinate	排尿 (はいにょう)
19. defecation	排便 (はいべん)
20. constipation	便秘 (べんぴ)

21. diarrhea	下痢 (げり)
22. sleep	睡眠 (すいみん)
23. eat	食べる (たべる)
24. walk	歩く (あるく)
25. run	走る (はしる)
26. laugh	笑う (わらう)
27. cry	泣く (なく)
28. speak	話す (はなす)
29. think	考える (かんがえる)
30. dream	夢を見る (ゆめをみる)
31. recall	思い出す (おもいだす)
32. childhood	幼年時代 (ようねんじだい)
33. adolescence	青年期 (せいねんき)
34. puberty	思春期 (ししゅんき)
35. adulthood	成人期 (せいじんき)
36. medical intern	医学研修生(いがくけんしゅうせい)
37. specialist	専門医 (せんもんい)
38. surgery	外科 (げか)
39. surgeon	外科医 (げかい)
40. receptionist	受付係 (うけつけがかり)

Medical Terms: Practice

Use the medical terms to complete the sentences.

1) The professor said I need to get more sleep because I ____________________ too much in class, and the sound is very disruptive.

2) ____________________ is a difficult time for adolescents because so many changes are happening in their bodies.

3) My mother always told me to ____________________ my food 30 times before I ____________________ .

4) The nurse asked me if I was constipated, but I told him it was the opposite——I had really bad ____________________ !

5) A person with a high ____________________ can convert food much faster than the average person.

6) Even though my sister is now in her 40s, she can still ____________________ being taken to the hospital when she was four years old.

7) Whenever I see delicious pizza, I always ____________________ .

8) Is it rude to ____________________ ____________________ in an elevator?

9) When a person has an asthma attack, it is very difficult to ____________________ .

10) The best ____________________ in the hospital will be performing the ____________________ tomorrow.

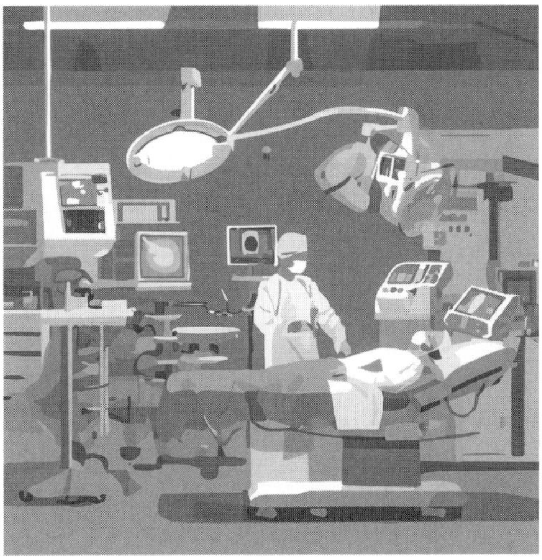

Grammar Review: Prepositions of Place

Look at these words and phrases:

at	behind	between	in
in front of	next to	on	opposite

These words and phrases show us where things or people are located. They are called **prepositions of place**. They are very important when working in a hospital or clinic because during emergencies, doctors, nurses, and other medical professionals must locate instruments, medicine, and machines very quickly. During an emergency, the faster medical professionals move, the better chance their patients have to survive.

Let's look at these prepositions of place in use:

1. Fushigi-chan is *at* the hospital.

2. Fushigi-chan is *behind* the desk.

3. Fushigi-chan is *between* the desks.

4. Fushigi-chan is *in* the desk.

5. Fushigi-chan is *in front of* the desk.

6. Fushigi-chan is *next to* the desk.

7. Fushigi-chan is *on* the desk.

8. Fushigi-chan is *opposite* the desk.

• Grammar Activity 1

Match the sentences (1-8) with the following pictures. Write the number next to the picture.

Picture A ______

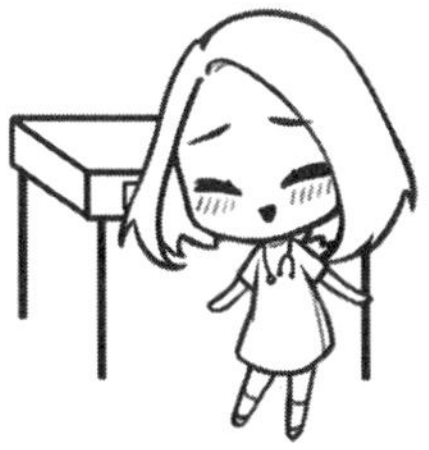

Picture B ______

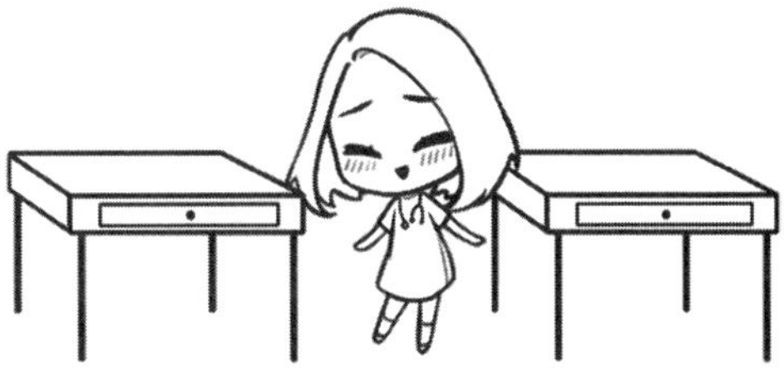

Picture C ______

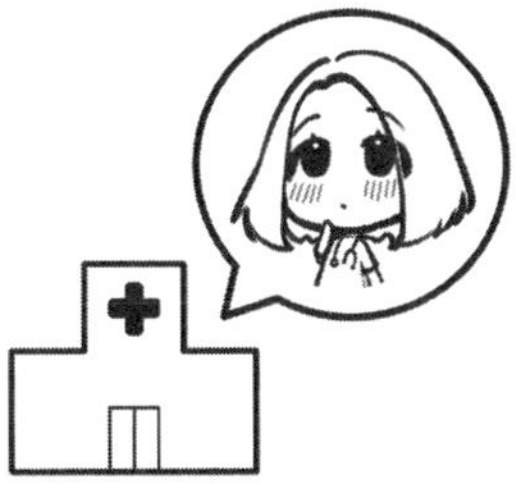

Picture D ______

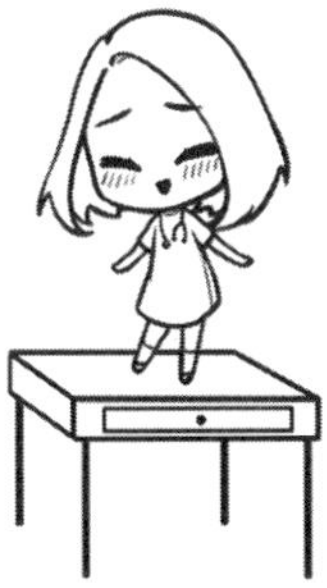

Picture E ______

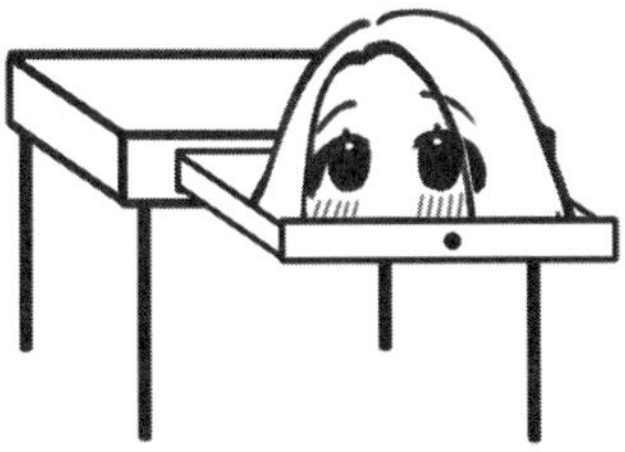

Picture F ______

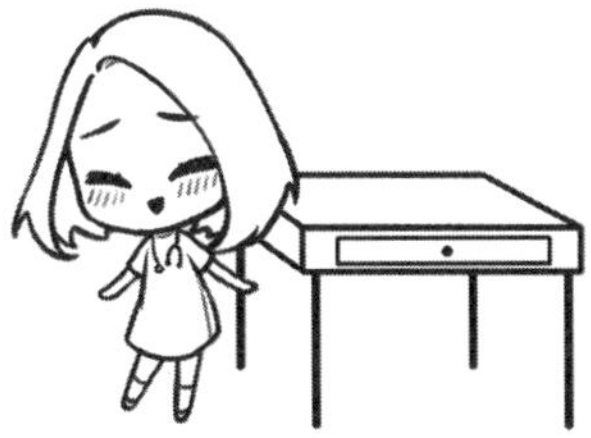

Picture G ______

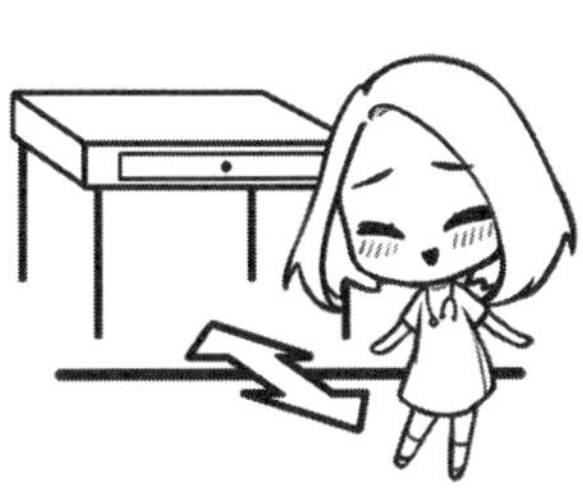

Picture H ______

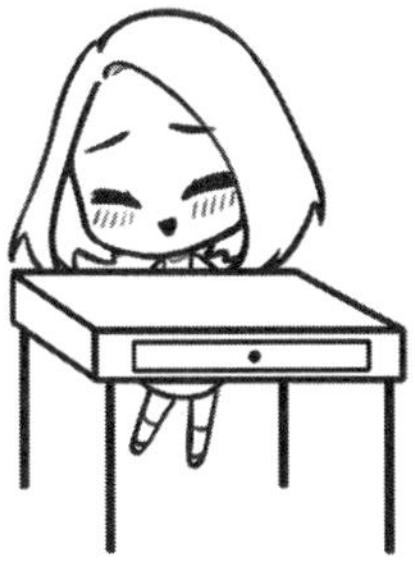

• Grammar Activity 2

Complete the sentences with the correct prepositions.

1. I'm sorry, but the doctor is currently ________ a conference ________ Canada.
2. The new ventilators are ________ the storage room ________ the hospital.
3. Your next appointment is ________ Tuesday morning ________ 9:45 a.m.
4. The nurse's station is located ________ ________ ________ the reception desk ________ the 4th floor.
5. The keys to the break room are ________ the table ________ the main door. Just turn around and you'll see them!

• Grammar Activity 3

After carefully looking at the picture of the waiting room, ask your partner questions about the location of the items. You can use the questions below or create your own. When you finish, switch roles! Write your answers to the questions in the space provided and check to make sure you used the correct prepositions. More than one answer may be possible.

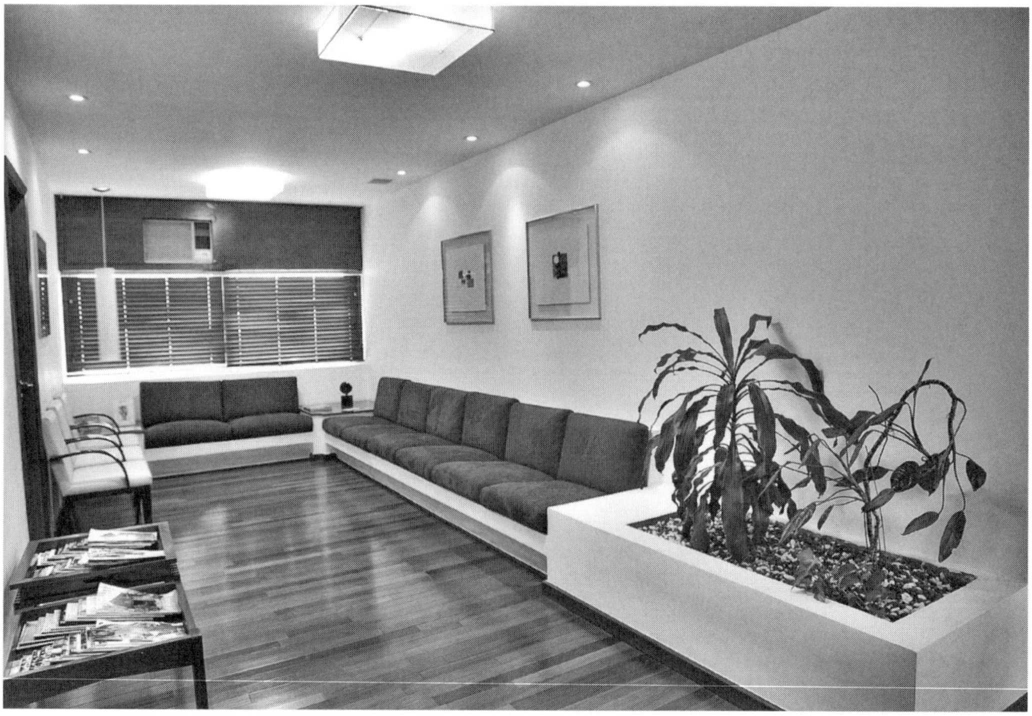

1. Where are the paintings?

____

2. Where are the plants?

____

3. Where are the white chairs?

____

4. Where are the magazines?

____

5. Where is the door?

____

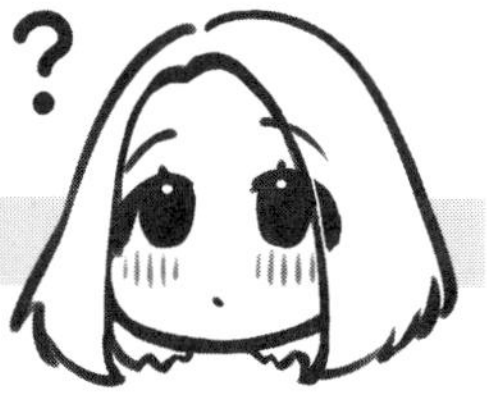

Reading with Fushigi-chan: Modern Lifestyles

Why do human beings get sick? Every year, millions of people get sick every day, from common colds to diarrhea. However, the recent COVID-19 pandemic has made many people wonder why the human body can't fight off every disease and virus.

It is true that human beings live much longer now compared to hundreds of years ago. That's because advances in medicine and technology have allowed us to stay healthier than ever before. So why can't our bodies fight off hay fever, the common cold, COVID-19, or cancer?

The answer is not simple, and many scientists are still trying to discover ways to bring an end to these ailments. One reason that should be considered is how life has changed over the last century. As mentioned, technology and medicine have extended life expectancies. However, modern life has also brought conveniences that have contributed to other ailments, such as obesity（肥満，ひまん）and diabetes（糖尿病，とうにょうびょう）.

One of these conveniences is fast food. Fast food chains, such as McDonalds and Mos Burger, and ready-to-eat meals that are sold in supermarkets and convenience stores have made life much easier to live because they adapt to busy lifestyles. These fast foods are also filled with high levels of calories, salt, and sugar, along with other things that the human body doesn't want or need.

Considering this, it is up to medical professionals to promote healthy lifestyles—exercising, eating healthier food, and maintaining stress levels. This is easier said than done, of course, given fast-paced lifestyles and demanding work schedules. It's also important to teach patients about the differences between infectious diseases (caused by bacteria and viruses) and non-infectious diseases (caused by factors such as a person's genetics, their lifestyle, and their environment) . Knowing this won't stop a pandemic, but it may be one key to keeping people healthy.

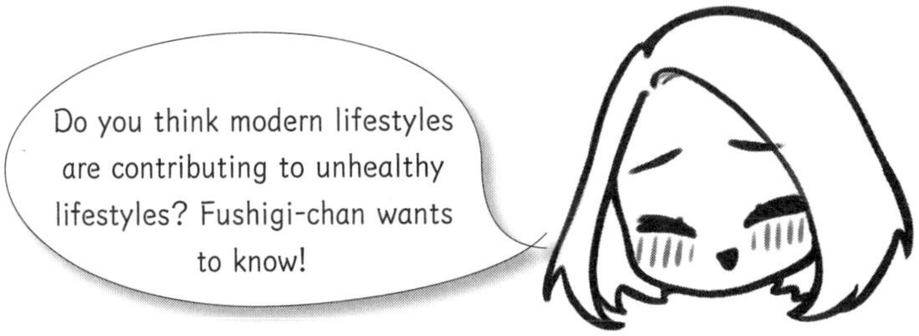

• Reading Activity 1

Fill in the blanks with the appropriate words.

1. Two things that have contributed to living longer are ________________ and ________________ .

2. Another word for an illness or other health issue, like obesity, is ________________ .

3. As a medical professional, you have an obligation to promote ________________ lifestyles.

4. Fast food and ________________ - ________________ - ________________ meals may be contributing to the body's inability to fight diseases.

5. Because of fast food and a lack of exercise, ________________ and ________________ are becoming widespread around the world.

• Reading Activity 2

Answer these questions related to the reading.

1. What is wrong with some ready-to-eat meals sold in supermarkets and convenience stores?

2. What are some changes that have increased life expectancy rates?

3. What are some reasons why humans become sick?

4. What are some differences between infectious and non-infectious diseases?

Writing Activity

When you become a medical professional, how will you promote a healthy lifestyle to your patients? Create a flyer（チラシ）that will explain your ideas in detail, and include pictures, charts, and statistics. For example, "According to the Center for Disease Control (2022) 41.9 % of adults in America are obese." You can use color pens, markers, and highlighters to make your flyer stand out. You can use the box below to write an outline or draft, but you should use a separate sheet of paper or poster board for the final version of the flyer.

After you're done, present your flyer to a small group or the entire class. Who has the most convincing flyer?

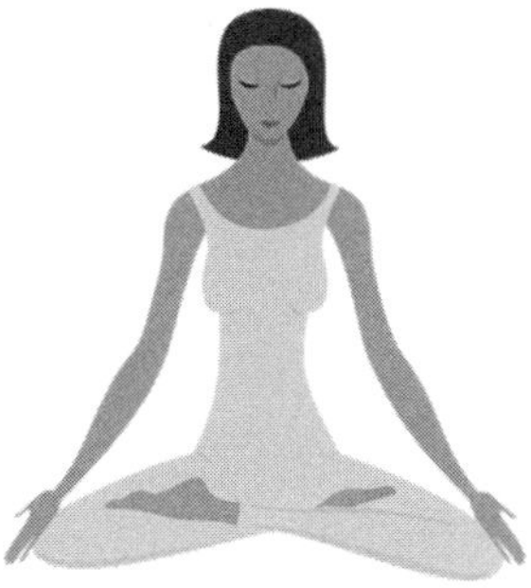

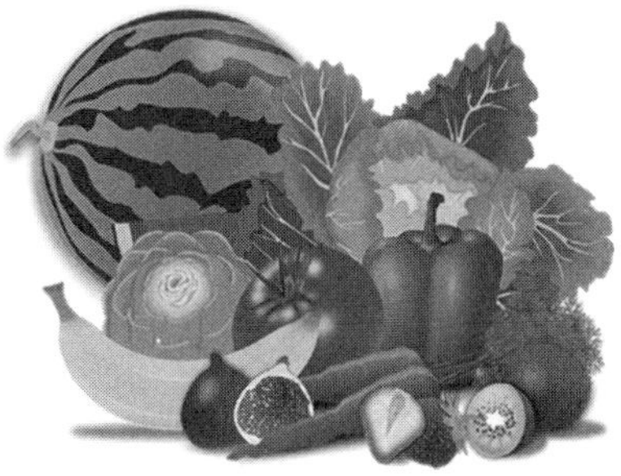

When you're finished, discuss the strong and weak areas. Which points do you think would help flyers stand out more to patients?

Listening Activity

Listen to a medical student talk about staying healthy while studying to become a doctor. Write the student's name and two things she does to stay mentally and physically healthy.

Speaker's Name: ____________________

1. ____

____

2. ____

____

Speaking Activity

Choose two countries—your own and another country you are familiar with. How do their lifestyles differ from each other? Are there certain health issues in one country but not in another? Is the medical situation the same (for example, everyone has free health insurance) or are there big differences (everyone must pay)? Use your electronic device to quickly research your chosen countries, and then write notes in the chart below. After you have finished, discuss the similarities and differences with a partner or the class.

My Country:	Another Country:
1	
2	
3	
4	
5	

Discussion Questions

1. Do you believe the average person in your country understands how their body functions? What information do you think might make people change their bad habits?
2. Do you think modern lifestyles are contributing to unhealthy lifestyles? How does your lifestyle reflect some of these modern changes? Would they be easy to give up (for example, fast food or your smartphone) ?
3. Do you think countries work together enough to make the world a better, safer, healthier place? How do they, or how do they not?

Speaking Strategies: General Speaking Skills, Part IV

In Unit 1, you learned about "Gestures for Focus." These are simple movements with your hands and arms that help the audience know what information (on the board, PowerPoint, etc.) you're talking about by drawing attention to that area. In this unit, we'll learn to use gestures for another important reason: "Gestures for Expression." These physical expressions help the audience understand key points you are talking about in your speech or presentation. Here are a few Gestures for Expression you can use in your speech or presentation, but remember that these gestures could also be used when you're engaged in a regular conversation with a friend, teacher or coworker!

Final Unit Assignment

Topic Utopia (ユートピア)

The idea of *utopia*, or a place where everything is perfect, has intrigued human beings for centuries. Does such a place exist, or can it ever exist? Medical professionals can't answer that question, but they can think about ways our world can change for the better.

Imagine tomorrow there are no more fast-food restaurants. All of them have suddenly disappeared. In addition, imagine there are no more smart phones. Those, too, have disappeared. How would you, as a medical professional, use this strange situation to improve the quality of healthcare to your patients? Would you appear on a talk show and promote certain changes? Would you create a new government program supporting exercise, regular health check-ups, and cancer screenings? What actions would you take to make people healthier and happier?

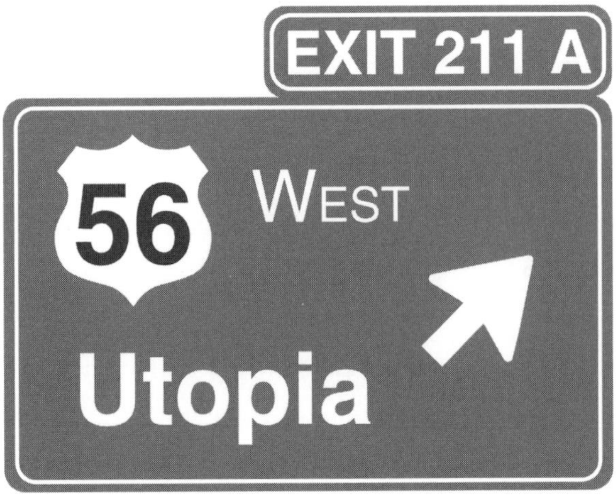

UNIT 5

Medical Histories

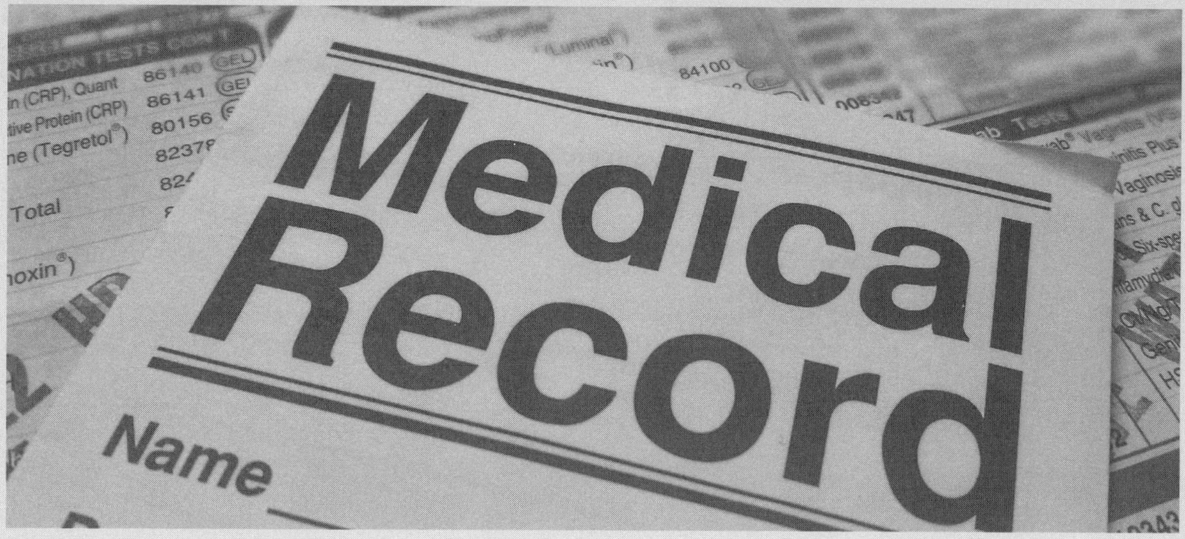

Medical Terms

1. medical history	既往歴 (きおうれき)
2. family history	家族歴 (かぞくれき)
3. case study	事例研究 (じれいけんきゅう)
4. date-of-birth (DOB)	生年月日 (せいねんがっぴ)
5. marital status	配偶者の有無 (はいぐうしゃのうむ)
6. occupation	職業 (しょくぎょう)
7. insurance	保険 (ほけん)
8. prescription	処方箋 (しょほうせん)
9. physical exam	診察 (しんさつ)
10. immunization	予防接種 (よぼうせっしゅ)
11. allergy	アレルギー
12. general practitioner (GP)	開業医 (かいぎょうい)
13. surgery	手術 (しゅじゅつ)
14. procedure	施術 (せじゅつ)
15. pain	痛み (いたみ)
16. headache	頭痛 (ずつう)
17. faint	気絶 (きぜつ)
18. blurry vision	視野のぼやけ (しやのぼやけ)
19. earache	耳痛 (じつう)
20. dizziness	目眩 (めまい)

21. shortness of breath	息切れ (いきぎれ)
22. sore throat	咽頭炎 (いんとうえん)
23. hemorrhage	出血 (しゅっけつ)
24. blood clot	血栓 (けっせん)
25. hypotension	低血圧 (ていけつあつ)
26. hypertension	高血圧 (こうけつあつ)
27. anorexia	食欲低下 (しょくよくていか)
28. heartburn	胸焼け (むねやけ)
29. stomachache	腹痛 (ふくつう)
30. nausea	吐き気 (はきけ)
31. vomit	吐き出す (はきだす)
32. pregnant	妊娠 (にんしん) した
33. weight gain	体重増加 (たいじゅうぞうか)
34. weight loss	体重減少 (たいじゅうげんしょう)
35. numb	麻痺 (まひ)
36. myalgia	筋肉痛 (きんにくつう)
37. cyst	嚢胞 (のうほう)
38. fatigue	疲労 (ひろう)
39. tumor	腫瘍 (しゅよう)
40. inflammation	炎症 (えんしょう)

Medical Terms: Practice

Find the meaning for each medical term.

1) vomit ____	•	• a. pain in a muscle or group of muscles
2) myalgia ____	•	• b. swelling
3) stomachache ____	•	• c. high blood pressure
4) dizziness ____	•	• d. loss of appetite
5) DOB ____	•	• e. birthday
6) fatigue ____	•	• f. tummy ache
7) anorexia ____	•	• g. unable to feel
8) numb ____	•	• h. tiredness
9) inflammation ____	•	• i. “the room is spinning”
10) hypertension ____	•	• j. throw up

Grammar Review: Comparative Adjectives

As you learned in a previous unit, adjectives describe nouns (people, places, and things). We use comparative adjectives when we want to compare two or more nouns.

Generally speaking, if an adjective has one or two syllables (音節, おんせつ), you can add *-er* + *than*.

Becoming a pharmacist is **hard*er* than** becoming a teacher.
The new hospital beds are **softer than** the old ones.

If an adjective ends in -y, add *-ier* + *than*.

Teaching is **eas*ier*** than healthcare.
Visiting a big hospital is **scarier than** small clinics.

For some adjectives, you have to double the consonants.

Men’s bodies are usually **bi*gger* than** women’s bodies.
Flatt*er* surfaces are **better** to work on **than** uneven surfaces.

If an adjective has two or more syllables, use *more* (adjective) *than*.

Hospitals are ***more*** important ***than*** convenience store.
The injection was ***more*** painful ***than*** the physical exam.

• Grammar Activity 1

Complete the chart with the correct form of comparative adjectives.

e.g. fast	faster (than)
strong	
healthy	
popular	
quick	
skinny	
good (note: this is a special comparative adjective)	(than)
bad (note: this is a special comparative adjective)	(than)

• Grammar Activity 2

Circle the correct comparative adjectives.

1. Elderly patients are (**difficulter / more difficult**) than children.
2. Bananas are (**more healthier / healthier**) than chocolate.
3. My chemistry professor is (**popularer / more popular**) than my anatomy professor.
4. The pain in my chest is getting (**worse / worst**) than the pain in my back.
5. This medical English textbook is (**best / better**) than the one we used last year!

• Grammar Activity 3

Rewrite the sentences and correct the comparative adjectives.

1. Doctors are more richer than teachers.
2. Is nursing a gooder job than being a surgeon?
3. I think the lights in Examination Room 7 are brightly than in Examination Room 12.

4. The physical therapist's vacation destination is more exoticer than the head nurse's destination.

____

5. The food in the faculty cafeteria is most deliciouser than the food in the student lounge.

____

Reading with Fushigi-chan: Medical Histories

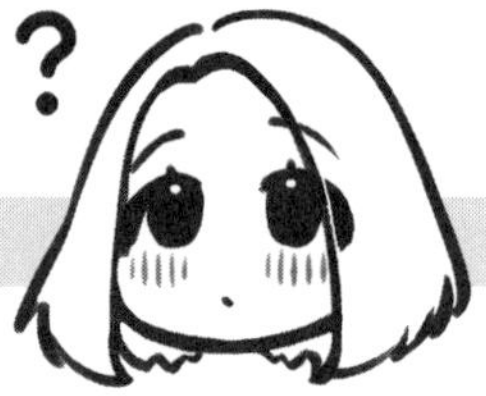

What is a medical history? Many 1st-year medical students might be confused about what exactly is a medical history, and that's because there are a few different parts that need to be considered.

First, we need to understand the purpose of taking a patient's medical history. By using the information from a medical history, doctors, nurses, and other medical specialists can make an initial diagnosis of what could be wrong with the patient. They can also see if the patient may be susceptible to future health issues.

A medical history is sometimes referred to as a past medical history (PMH) , a family history or a case history. Let's look at each one and talk about what is involved.

A past medical history usually asks patients for information about:

- past illnesses, including childhood illnesses
- immunization history
- accidents
- injuries
- past surgeries
- past and current medications
- allergies to food and medication

For female patients, it is important to also ask about any pregnancies in the past, if they are currently pregnant or think they might be pregnant, and any issues like miscarriages and abortions.

A family history asks about information related to the patient's family—the patient, his or her spouse or partner, and their biological children. This is known as a "nuclear family," but there are other types of families, as well (for example, single-parent families). The medical history of the patient's extended family—the parents, aunts, uncles, and so on—is also important because this can reveal any diseases that may be inherited (遺伝，いでん).

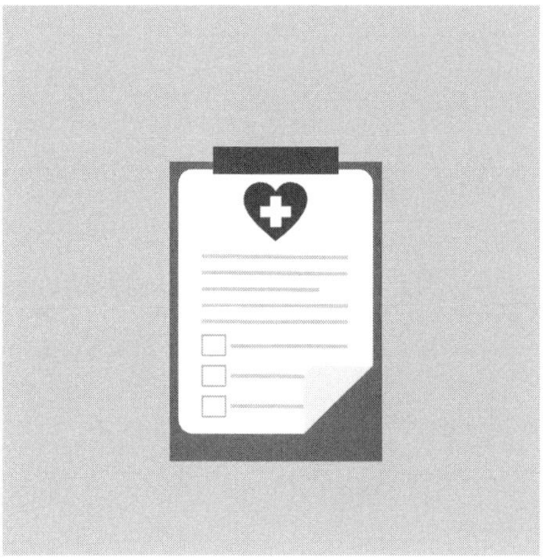

Although some may consider family histories, past medical histories and case histories to be the same, a case history can be seen as containing more information. Not only does a case history have all the information from a past medical history and family history, but it also has the presenting problem (the reason the patient came to visit the doctor), results of a physical exam the doctor or nurse performed, as well as results from any tests conducted on the patient (for example, an x-ray performed by an x-ray technician, or a blood test performed by a phlebotomist). Using all this information, a doctor or a team of doctors, nurses, and specialists can decide what the cause (s) of the presenting complaint may be and what treatment (s) could help. Treatment could include physical therapy, medications, surgery, or a combination of all of these.

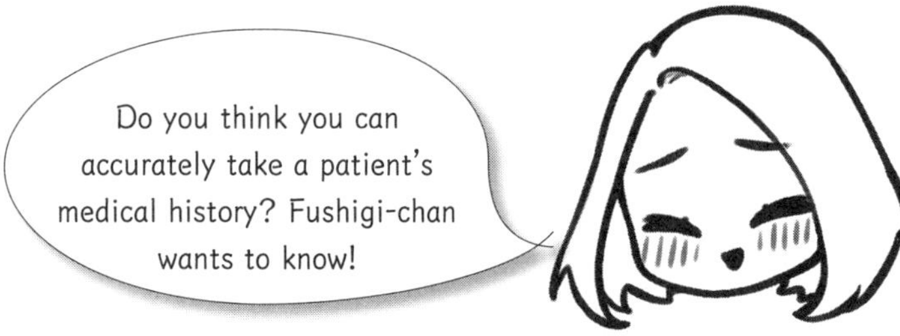

• Reading Activity 1

Answer these questions about histories.

1. What are all the parts of a past medical history?

____

____

2. Why are medical histories important?

____

____

3. What are the differences between a past medical history and a family history?

____

____

4. What does a case history contain?

____

____

5. What do medical professionals do with all the information in a case history?

____

____

• Reading Activity 2

Match the words and phrases in the box below to their meaning. If you're not sure of the meaning, find the words or phrases in the reading section and try to figure out their meaning from the words around them.

miscarriage	physical exam	nuclear family
susceptible	immunization	

1. ______________ spontaneous abortion
2. ______________ a couple and their dependent children
3. ______________ making a person immune to infection through inoculation
4. ______________ medical examination to determine a patient's health
5. ______________ likely to be harmed by something

Writing Activity

Fill out the Medical History form below. To make the activity more interesting, write information that is not true for sections like *Allergies* and *Past Surgeries*, , For example you can write “Allergies: Peanuts; Past Surgeries: rhinoplasty.” Maybe you don’t have any allegies and have never had surgery, but now you have more information to help you practice medical English.

Medical History

Patient’s Name:

DOB:

Name of GP:

Date of last physical:

Immunization record? _____ Y _____ N

Health insurance? _____ Y _____ N

Past illnesses (procedure and date) :

Accidents (type of accident and date) :

Injuries (type of injury and date) :

Past surgeries (procedure and date) :

Past medications used (name and dosage, if known) :

Current medications used (name and dosage) :

Allergies:

When you’re finished, share what you wrote with a partner. You can also use this form for the **Speaking Activity** below?

Listening Activity

Listen to a nurse talk to a potential patient. Since he is not a patient yet, the nurse is not taking a formal medical history. She is only asking the man questions about his current status, medical history, and presenting problem. While you listen, complete the doctor's notes below.

Patient's name:

DOB:

Marital status:

Children:

Occupation:

C/o:

Current symptoms:

How often:

Past medical history:

Family history:

Current medications:

Speaking Activity

With a partner, take turns asking each other questions in order to get the information needed to complete a medical history. For example, to get your partner's name, you would ask, "What is your name?" or "Full name, please?" For last physical, you could ask, "When was your last physical exam?" or "Do you remember the date of your last physical?"

Write your partner's answers in the **Medical History** form on the next page. Be sure to write the correct information! If you're not sure of an answer, say, "Pardon?" or "Could you repeat that, please?"

Medical History

Patient's Name:

DOB:

Name of GP:

Date of last physical:

Immunization record? ______ Y ______ N

Health insurance? ______ Y ______ N

Past illnesses (procedure and date) :

Accidents (type of accident and date) :

Injuries (type of injury and date) :

Past surgeries (procedure and date) :

Past medications used (name and dosage, if known) :

Current medications used (name and dosage) :

Allergies:

When you're finished, present your medical history to the class!

Discussion Questions

1. In your home country, what questions are asked during a medical history? Who usually takes the medical history—a doctor, nurse, office staff or someone else?
2. How would you rate the healthcare system in your country? What could be done to improve the system for all groups (children, adults, elderly) ?

3. Can you think of any questions that are asked during a medical history that may be embarrassing or offensive to a person from a different country than the one you're currently in? Think of one or two example questions, and change them so they might not be so embarrassing or offensive.

Speaking Strategies: Cultural Gestures

In the previous units, you learned a lot about using your body, eyes, voice, and hands to send various messages to your audience. In this unit, we will look at how gestures may be used within and across different cultures.

Final Unit Assignment

Topic Majority vs. Minority

In a group, the minority is the smaller number of people who share the same idea or opinion. The majority is the larger group of people who share the same idea or opinion.

Split the classroom into two groups—one smaller than the other. For example, if the class size is 30, one group could be 8-10 people (the minority) and the rest would be the majority group.

The **minority group** will create ten (10) changes that they want to make in the hospital. For example, faster job promotions, more scholarships for medical students, and free housing for all students and faculty.

The **majority group** will have to come up with reasons to oppose each request.

20 minutes: Preparation time for each group.

10 minutes: Debate (The **minority group** presents one change, followed by a rebuttal by the **majority group**. Continue until all changes are presented and challenged) .

10 minutes: Classroom discussion. How did you feel being part of each group?

Remember: The goal is not to highlight how unfair majority groups can be to minority groups or to argue and "point fingers" (i.e., blame each other) , but to go through a debate in order to understand both sides of a group dispute. You don't have to agree with one side or the other—you simply have to gain a better understanding of group dynamics.

UNIT 6

Physical Exams

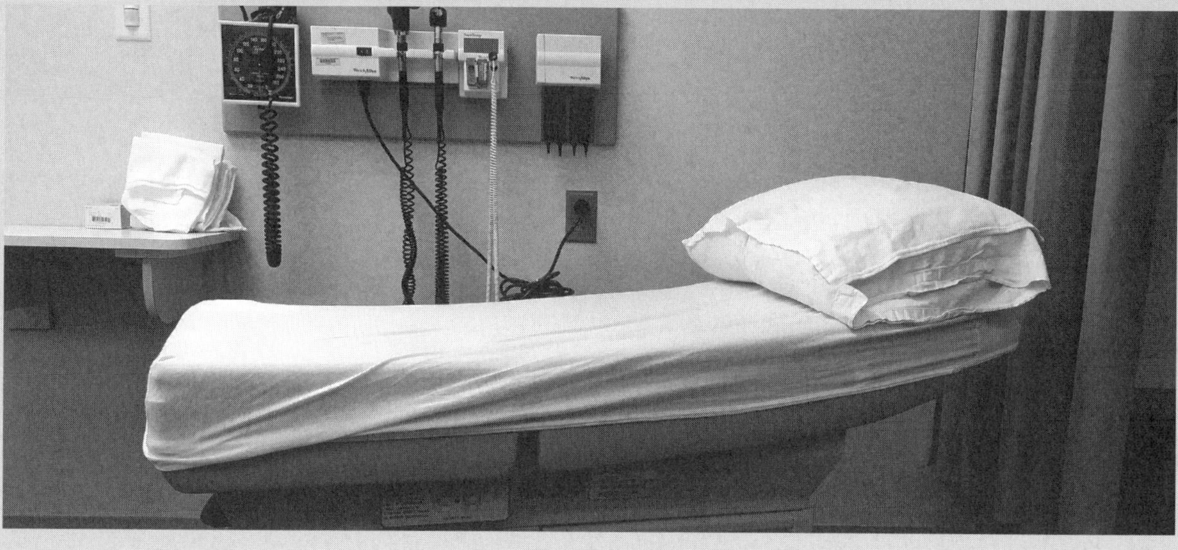

Medical Terms

1. critical condition	危篤状態 (きとくじょうたい)
2. infectious disease	感染症 (かんせんしょう)
3. benign	良性 (りょうせい)
4. malignant	悪性 (あくせい)
5. metastasis	転移 (てんい)
6. remission	寛解 (かんかい)
7. recurrence	再発 (さいはつ)
8. congenital	先天性 (せんてんせい)
9. cure	治癒 (ちゆ)
10. heal	治る (なおる)
11. remedy	治療 (ちりょう)
12. aggravate	悪化させる (あっかさせる)
13. patient	患者 (かんじゃ)
14. body temperature	体温 (たいおん)
15. prognosis	予後 (よご)
16. stable condition	小康状態 (しょうこうじょうたい)
17. recover	回復 (かいふく)
18. initial stage	初期段階 (しょきだんかい)
19. convalescent stage	回復期 (かいふくき)
20. progressive stage	進行期 (しんこうき)
21. terminal stage	末期 (まっき)

22. person who has tested positive	陽性者 (ようせいしゃ)
23. person who has tested negative	陰性者 (いんせいしゃ)
24. mild case	軽い症例 (かるいしょうれい)
25. severe case	ひどい症例(ひどいしょうれい)
26. rare case	まれな症例(まれなしょうれい)
27. persistent	持続的 (じぞくてき)
28. previous disease	既往症 (きおうしょう)
29. antigen	抗原 (こうげん)
30. antibody	抗体 (こうたい)
31. auscultation	聴診 (ちょうしん)
32. biopsy	生検 (せいけん)
33. bone exam	骨検査 (こつけんさ)
34. blood pressure	血圧 (けつあつ)
35. blood count	血球数 (けっきゅうすう)
36. blood coagulation	血液凝固 (けつえきぎょうこ)
37. glucose	グルコース
38. blood type	血液型 (けつえきがた)
39. blood sample	血液標本(けつえきひょうほん)
40. psychosomatic	心因性 (しんいんせい)

Medical Terms: Practice

Circle the words that patients would use to describe these medical terms.

1) recover	a. get better	b. get worse	c. mild
2) infectious	a. infestation	b. dirty	c. contagious
3) diffuse	a. widespread	b. area	c. get better
4) aggravate	a. allow	b. make worse	c. grind
5) auscultation	a. seeing	b. feeling	c. listening
6) glucose	a. blood	b. blood sugar	c. blood level
7) persistent	a. sweaty	b. annoying	c. constant
8) prognosis	a. prediction	b. cancer	c. assurance
9) benign	a. kind	b. harmless	c. harmful
10) malignant	a. cancerous	b. evil	c. able to catch

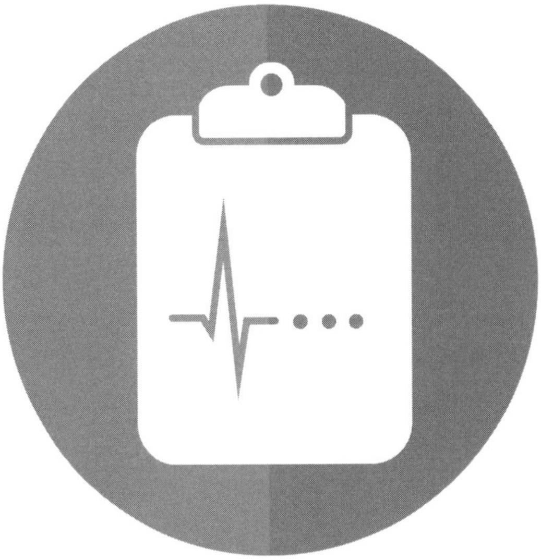

Grammar Review: Prefixes

Prefixes are important parts of words because they give you clues to the word's meaning. Prefixes are letters that we can add to the beginning of words to make a new word and change their meaning. Here are ten common prefixes and how they change the meanings of some words.

Prefix	Base word	New word and meaning
a-	moral	**amoral**: lacking morals
auto-	mobile	**automobile**: a car
co-	worker	**coworker**: a person who works with you
dis-	appear	**disappear**: to stop being visible
extra-	curricular	**extracurricular**: done outside of the regular school schedule
im-	possible	**impossible**: not able to be done
inter-	personal	**interpersonal**: a person's relationships with other people
intra-	personal	**intrapersonal**: relating to the self
over-	stimulate	**overstimulate**: stimulate too much
un-	able	**unable**: not able to do something

Medical terms are difficult to learn, but if you know the meaning of the prefixes, you have a good idea about the meaning of the entire word. Here are ten common prefixes found in medical terms.

Medical term prefix	Meaning	Example word / 日本語
aut-	self	autopsy/ 検視 (けんし)
dia-	through; across; omplete	diagnosis/ 診断 (しんだん)
dys-	not working well; not functioning normally	dysfunction/ 機能不全 (きのうふぜん)
endo-	within	endoscopy/ 内視鏡 (ないしきょう)
hyper-	too much; more than normal	hyperthyroidism/ 甲状腺機能亢進症 (こうじょうせんきのうこうしんしょう)
hypo-	too little; less than normal	hypothyroidism/ 甲状腺機能低下症 (こうじょうせんきのうこうしんていかしょう)
inter-	between	interstitial/ 間質性 (かんしつせい)
mal-	bad	malabsorption/ 吸収不良症候群 (きゅうしゅうふりょうしょうこうぐん)
peri-	around; about	pericardium/ 心膜 (しんまく)
sub-	under; below	subcutaneous/ 皮下 (ひか)
trans-	across	transdermal patch/ 貼付剤 (ちょうふざい)

As mentioned in the introduction, you should invest in a medical terminology book.

• Grammar Activity 1

Circle the best answer for each question or statement.

1. The prefix "pre" can be used at the beginning of which word?

   [a. determine b. choose c. medical d. sleep]

2. The prefix "poly," like in the word polyglot (-glot means *tongue or speaking and writing in a language*) means:

   [a. more b. any c. many d. some]

3. Which of the following is a prefix?

   [a. tion b. co c. ness d. ity]

4. Choose the correct prefix to add to the word medication to make it mean "too much medication."

   [a. under b. co c. hyper d. over]

5. Choose the correct prefix to add to the word regular to make it mean "not regular."

   [a. ir b. un c. non d. dis]

• Grammar Activity 2

Use the prefixes in **Activity 1** to complete the sentences.

1. Theme parks are ___________ stop fun because there are so many things to do!
2. The hospital is really ___________ staffed, so patients have to wait a long time. They need to hire more doctors and nurses.
3. When a patient has multiple cysts, it is referred to as ___________ cystic.
4. When the professor asked for a larger office, the university immediately ___________ approved of the request.
5. My job is very stressful, but I love my ___________ workers, so I decided not to quit.

• Grammar Activity 3

Choose the correct prefix to make a medical term. After you choose the prefix, write the entire word below and then check the meaning in your dictionary.

1. sub •	• a. ism
2. aut •	• b. tension
3. peri •	• c. entery
4. hypo •	• d. lingual
5. dys •	• e. umbilical

word		meaning
1. ____________	:	____
2. ____________	:	____
3. ____________	:	____
4. ____________	:	____
5. ____________	:	____

Reading with Fushigi-chan: The Hippocratic Oath

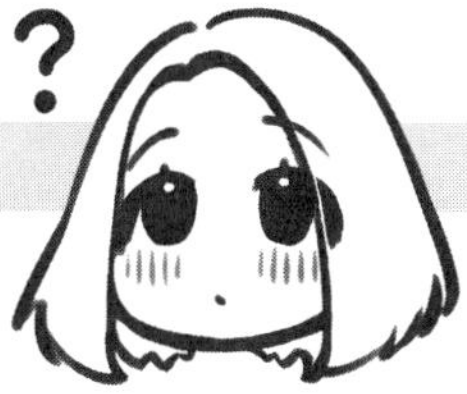

Have you ever thought about the history of physical exams? When did medical professionals start to do them? What tools did they use to examine the body?

During your medical studies, perhaps you have learned about or at least heard of Hippocrates. He was a Greek physician who lived from 460 B.C. to 370 B.C. and is usually referred to as the "Father of Medicine" because he did so much to establish medicine as a field. There is a lot of information on Hippocrates, his work, and his influence on modern medicine, and while it is difficult to know what is actually true because he lived so long ago, we do know many things about him.

Most importantly, Hippocrates was the first person to believe diseases happened naturally, instead of believing bad things happened to people because of magic or gods. This belief led to progress in the field of medicine, including the practice of giving people physical exams. Hippocrates is one of several prominent physicians credited with the physical exam.

The tools used for physical exams and other medical procedures are very similar to what medical professionals use now. Physical exams require medical professionals to *observe* (look) , *palpate* (touch) , *percuss* (tap) , and *auscultate* (listen) , and these can be done without tools, although a stethoscope is typically used when listening to the sounds of the body. Tools, such as scalpels, hooks, forceps, and needles were also used, along with bandages, threads, and various oils and ointments. Medical procedures were most likely extremely painful in ancient times, but nowadays physical exams and other procedures often involve very little pain.

If you are studying to become a doctor, you will probably be required to take the Hippocratic Oath—an oath of ethics—although it is usually taken with other modern oaths made by national medical associations. If you are studying to be a nurse, you will probably be asked to take some form of The Nightingale Pledge, which is not really an oath, but more of a promise to do your best and not harm patients. Other areas in the medical field have similar oaths or promises, but this depends on the field and the country where one is practicing.

One thing is certain, though— Hippocrates worked very hard to practice and teach medicine. He truly is the Father of Medicine!

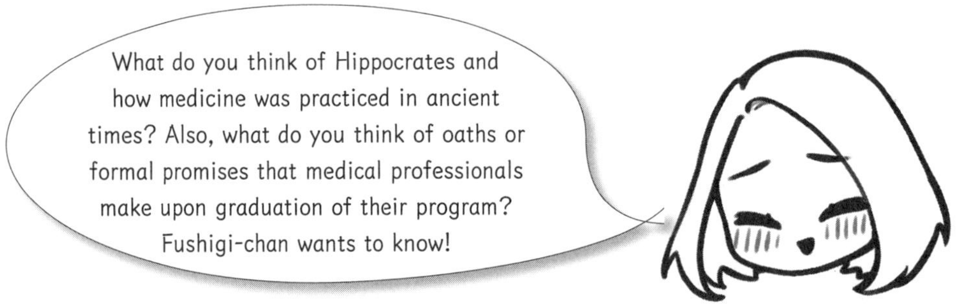

• Reading Activity 1

Circle (T) if the statement is true or (F) if the statement is false.

1. The practice of physical exams happened very recently. (T・F)
2. Hippocrates lived in Greece from 460 B.C. to 370 B.C. (T・F)
3. Hippocrates believed disease happened naturally and divinely. (T・F)
4. Hippocrates is known as the Grandfather of Medicine. (T・F)
5. Everything we know about Hippocrates is 100% true. (T・F)

• Reading Activity 2

Fill in the blanks with the appropriate words.

1. Another word for palpate is ________________ .
2. In ancient times, many people believed diseases happened because of ________________ or ________________ .
3. Tools, such as ________________ , ________________ , ________________ , and ________________ were used in ancient medical practices.
4. A stethoscope is used to listen, or ________________ , to the inside of the patient's body.
5. Many medical institutions still have graduates take the ________________ ________________ , although more modern ethical oaths are also used.

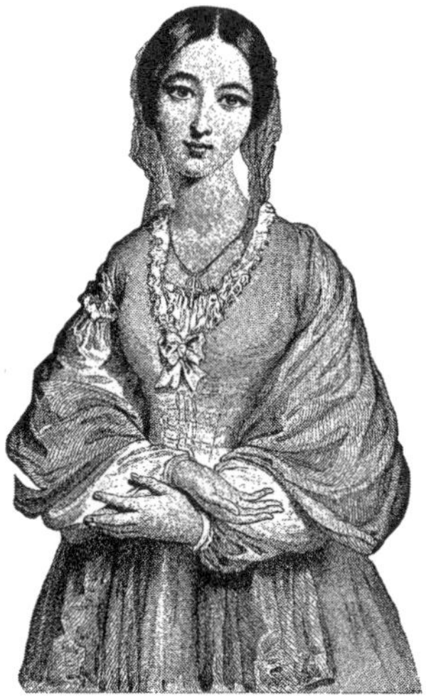

Florence Nightingale

Writing Activity

What happens during a physical exam? Work with a partner, and write as many steps as possible in the box below. Write down the instructions that medical professionals give patients during each step. For example, when listening to a patient's chest with a stethoscope, a doctor or nurse might say, "Take a deep breath in, hold it for ten seconds, and then breathe out."

You can also draw pictures of any medical instruments or machines used during physical exams, like a stethoscope.

When you're finished, share your writing with a partner or the class.

Listening Activity

Listen to a doctor giving different instructions to a patient during a physical exam. While you listen, fill in the missing information in the excerpts below.

1. I'm going to draw some blood from your arm, so ______________________________
____?

2. I want you to ______________________________
and then hold it for three seconds.

3. Now I want you to ______________________________ .

4. Now I want you to ______________________________ .

5. I'm going to apply some ______________________________ ,
so tell me if you feel any pain.

6. Please ____________________ forwards. Great. Do you feel any pain?

7. Could you ____________________? OK, now put your arm back down.

8. I'd like for you to ______________________________ .

9. Let me know if you ______________________________ .

10. Now I'm going to ____________________, so would you mind
____________________ and sitting on the examination table?

Speaking Activity

With a partner, use the script from the previous Listening Activity section to role-play a doctor or nurse giving a patient instructions during a physical exam. You can use the information from the activity or create a new situation using your own ideas or ideas from a previous unit. When you're finished, you and your partner can switch roles.

Discussion Questions

1. In your home country, is the Hippocratic Oath still a part of medical education? What are your thoughts on the oath? Do you think it's still relevant or should a new oath be adopted?

2. Think about your last physical exam. What parts of the exam went well? For example, "It didn't hurt when the nurse drew my blood." What parts could have been improved? For example, "The doctor could have explained the eye exam better."

3. Discuss what you know (or would like to know more) about psychosomatic illness (心因性, しんいんせい). What physical symptoms could manifest (come from) a mental or emotional event?

Speaking Strategies: Debate Skills, Part I

In **Unit 5**, you had the opportunity to be involved in a formal debate—"formal" meaning there were two sides, and it was organized in some way. In this section, we will begin to look at some basic debate skills.

First, what is a debate, and why are debate skills important? A debate is not a passionate fight or an angry challenge, but a controlled, respectful argument for or against a certain issue that is usually viewed as controversial in some way. People who are in a debate use reasons, examples, and statistics to prove their point in order to persuade a group of people who are judging the debate, or audience members. What differentiates debates and regular arguments? There are rules that debaters must follow.

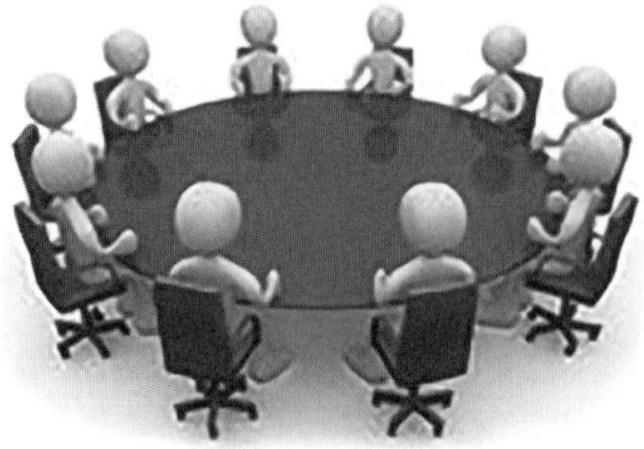

Final Unit Assignment

Topic To be or not to be... a medical professional

Before starting the assignment, view your reasons for wanting to become a medical professional in **Unit 1**. When all participants are ready, choose from one of the options below.

<u>Option A—Roundtable Discussion</u>

The entire class should sit in a circle (the "roundtable") so everyone is facing each other. When everyone is seated with their notes, have a conversation about the reasons for becoming a medical professional.

Make sure that each person speaks at least once!

<u>Option B—Debate</u>

Divide the class into two teams. Decide which team encourages students to become medical professionals and which team discourages students to become medical professionals. Use the chart from the Speaking Strategies to guide your response times. Remember that you don't have to really *believe* "all students should study medicine." This is just an exercise to practice expressing ideas and opinions in a debate format.

<u>Option C—Reflection Paper</u>

Write about both sides of this argument: Why do some students decide to go to medical school and why do other students decide to study a major that is not related to the medical field? Write a one-page reflection essay and prepare to discuss what you wrote.

UNIT 7

Other Types of Exams

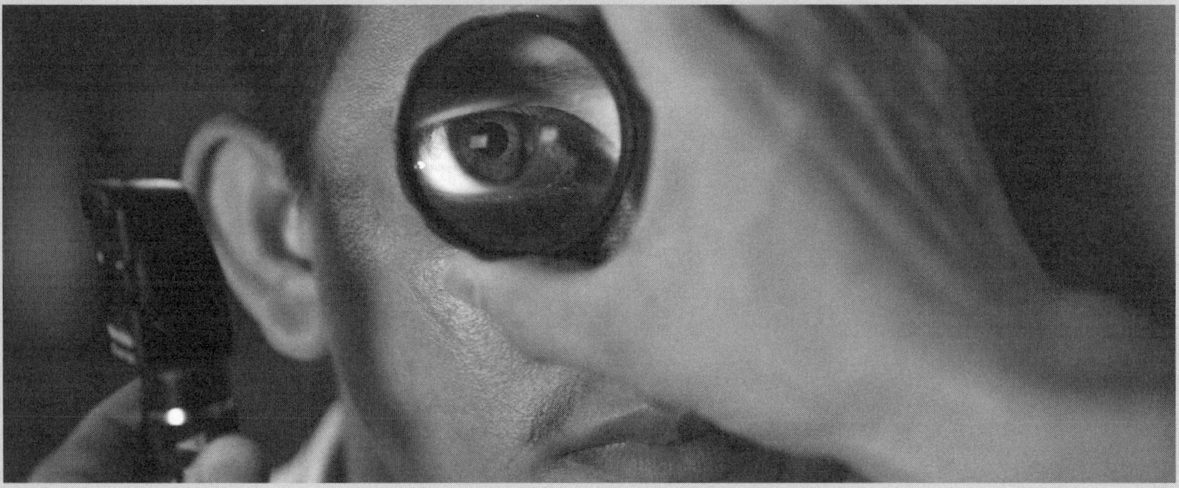

Medical Terms

1. X-ray test	X 線検査 (えっくすせんけんさ)
2. Computerized Tomography scan	コンピューター連動断層撮影 (れんどうだんそうさつえい)
3. brain wave	脳波 (のうは)
4. electrocardiogram	心電図 (しんでんず)
5. gastroscopy	胃カメラ検査 (いかめらけんさ)
6. mammogram	乳房 X 線撮影 (にゅうぼうえっくすせんさつえい)
7. ultrasound	超音波 (ちょうおんぱ)
8. pelvic exam	骨盤検査 (こつばんけんさ)
9. pap smear	子宮頸がん検査 (しきゅうけいがんけんさ)
10. digital exam	指診 (ししん)
11. rectal exam	直腸診 (ちょくちょうしん)
12. stool exam	便検査 (べんけんさ)
13. barium exam	バリウム検査 (けんさ)
14. endoscopy	内視鏡検査 (ないしきょうけんさ)
15. Magnetic Resonance Imaging	磁気共鳴映像法 (じききょうめいえいぞうほう)
16. positive	陽性の (ようせいの)
17. negative	陰性の (いんせいの)
18. abnormal level	異常値 (いじょうち)
19. angiography	血管造影
20. bronchoscopy	気管支鏡検査 (きかんしきょうけんさ)

21. catheter	カテーテル
22. hearing exam	聴力検査 (ちょうりょくけんさ)
23. pathology test	病理検査 (びょうりけんさ)
24. liver function test	肝機能検査 (かんきのうけんさ)
25. lung capacity test	肺活量検査(はいかつりょうけんさ)
26. ophthalmoscopic exam	検眼鏡検査(けんがんきょうけんさ)
27. tuberculosis test	結核検査 (けっかくけんさ)
28. urinalysis	尿検査 (にょうけんさ)
29. reflex test	反射テスト (はんしゃてすと)
30. vision test	視力検査 (しりょくけんさ)
31. pulse rate	脈拍数 (みゃくはくすう)
32. sputum test	喀痰検査 (かくたんけんさ)
33. tissue exam	組織検査 (そしきけんさ)
34. serology test	血清検査 (けっせいけんさ)
35. red blood cell count	赤血球数 (せっけっきゅうすう)
36. white blood cell count	白血球数 (はっけっきゅうすう)
37. erythrocyte sedimentation rate	赤血球沈降速度 (せっけっきゅうちんこうそくど), 赤沈 (せきちん)
38. cholesterol test	コレステロール検査 (けんさ)
39. Human Immuno-deficiency Virus test	ヒト免疫不全ウイルス検査 (ひとめんえきふぜんういるすけんさ)
40. Intelligence Test	知能テスト (ちのうてすと)

Medical Terms: Practice

Match the medical terms (1-10) to their acronyms (a-j).

1) blood pressure (from Unit 6) •	• a. TB
2) Computerized Tomography •	• b. IQ Test
3) electrocardiography •	• c. RBC
4) Intelligence Test •	• d. MRI
5) erythrocyte sedimentation rate •	• e. BP
6) Magnetic Resonance Imagining •	• f. EKG
7) tuberculosis •	• g. WBC
8) red blood cell count •	• h. CT
9) white blood cell count •	• i. HIV
10) Human Immuno-deficiency Virus •	• j. ESR

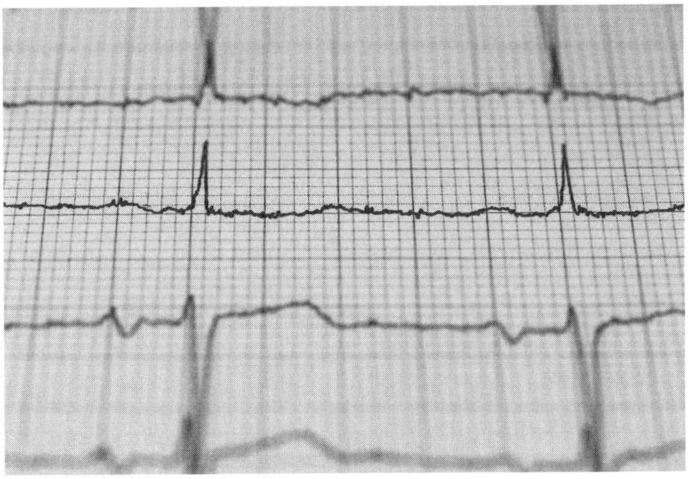

Grammar Review: Suffixes

Suffixes, like prefixes (see **Unit 6**) are also important parts of words that can help you understand their meaning. As you recall, prefixes are letters that are added to the beginning of a word to make a new word and change its meaning. Suffixes have the same function except they appear at the end of words. Suffixes can also change many types of words. There are suffixes for nouns (for example, reader) , adjectives (for example, readable) , and verbs (for example, generalize) . Lastly, although there is a list of suffixes to memorize, it is important to understand a word's meaning by its context (in other words, what comes before and after the word) . By understanding the gist (the general meaning) of the sentence, you will have a better idea of the word's meaning.

Here are ten common suffixes and how they change the meanings of some words.

Suffix	Base word	New word and meaning
-ance	process of	**clearance**: the process of getting rid of something
-er	a person who	**teacher**: person who teaches
-ist	a person who	**dentist**: a doctor who specializes in teeth and gums
-ity	quality of	**inactivity**: not active
-ment	condition of	**argument**: a fight or dispute
-ness	state of being	**happiness**: state of being happy
-or	a person who	**doctor**: a person who practices medicine
-ship	position held	**internship**: a job that is usually unpaid and provides training and experience
-sion	state of being	**transmission**: the process of transferring or passing on something
-tion	state of being	**operation**: performing surgery on someone

The above suffixes are for nouns, but there are many more suffixes that are commonly used for adjectives, such as -cal (for example, *medical*) and -able (for example, *operable*) , and for verbs, such as -ate (for example, *regulate*) and -ify (for example, *rectify*) . Please connect your study of suffixes (and prefixes) to the grammar lesson on nouns and adjectives in **Unit 2**.

As you just learned, if you know the meaning of the suffix, then you can have a good idea about the meaning of an entire word. Medical terms are, of course, difficult, but understanding suffixes will also help you a lot when trying to remember their meaning. Here are ten common suffixes found in medical terms.

Medical term suffix	Meaning	Example word / 日本語
-ectomy	removal of	hysterectomy / 子宮摘出（しきゅうてきしゅつ）
-gram	picture	interstitial / 間質性（かんしつせい）
-iatry	field of medical practice	podiatry / 足病学（そくびょうがく）
-iatrist	specialist in a field of medicine	psychiatrist / 精神科医（せいしんかい）
-itis	inflammation	hepatitis / 肝炎（かんえん）
-ology	study of	oncology / 腫瘍学（しゅようがく）
-ologist	person who specializes in a specific field, disease, or part of the body	radiologist / 放射線科医（ほうしゃせんかい）
- (o) tomy	act of making a cut or incision	anatomy / 解剖学（かいぼうがく）
-plasty	repairing or modifying the shape of	rhinoplasty / 隆鼻術（りゅうびじゅつ）
-stomy	act of creating an opening in	colostomy / 人工肛門造設術（じんこうこうもんぞうせつじゅつ）

As mentioned in Unit 6, you should study a medical terminology book in order to get a deep understanding of all the parts of medical terms—the prefixes, roots, and suffixes. By understanding the three parts and memorizing common prefixes and suffixes, you will be able to have a general understanding of many medical terms.

• Grammar Activity 1

Circle the best answer for each question or statement.

1. Which one can the suffix "otomy" be used at the end?

   [a. lob b. hyper c. psych d. hyster]

2. The suffix "-able," like in the word *operable*, means:

   [a. like b. act of creating an opening c. operate d. having the means to do something]

3. Which of the following is a suffix?

   [a. leuk b. co c. hypo d. ity]

4. Choose the correct suffix to add to the word tonsil to make it mean "inflammation of the tonsils."

   [a. tonsilectomy b. tonsilscopy c. tonsilitis d. tonsilstomy]

5. Choose the correct suffix to add to the word *trachea* to make it mean "opening in the trachea in order to insert a breathing tube."

[a. plasty b. otomy c. oscopy d. ectomy]

• Grammar Activity 2

Use the prefixes in **Grammar Review** to complete the sentences.

1. I'm considering rhino __________ . I think my nose is too big!
2. In order to access the patient's brain, a crani __________ was performed, which is a surgical cutting of the skull.
3. After we finish the nursing program, we have to go through a two-year intern __________ . This will provide us with lots of great experience!
4. Rika had a strong passion to help young women, so she decided to specialize in gynec __________ .
5. The doctor must be very careful when performing the eye surgery, otherwise they may cause blind __________ in a patient.

• Grammar Activity 3

Choose the correct suffix to make a medical term. After you choose the suffix, write the entire word below and then check the meaning in your dictionary.

1. blepharo	•	•	a. iatrist
2. hyster	•	•	b. plasty
3. pod	•	•	c. gram
4. gingiv	•	•	d. itis
5. electrocardio	•	•	e. ectomy

	word		meaning
1.	__________	:	______________________________
2.	__________	:	______________________________
3.	__________	:	______________________________
4.	__________	:	______________________________

5. ______________ : ____

Reading with Fushigi-chan: Medical Exams

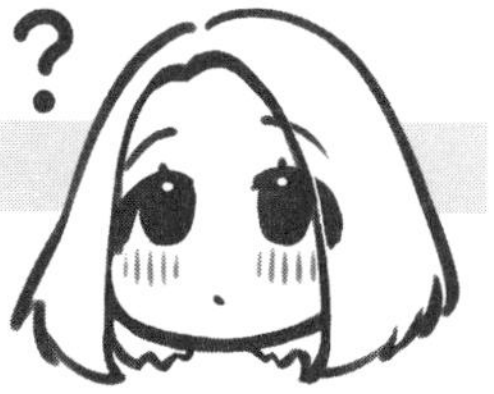

In the last unit, we looked at physical exams, including the history of the physical and some of the tools and actions used to perform one. There are many other medical procedures that are almost as common as a physical and are performed every year to millions of people in hospitals and clinics around the world.

While the physical exam is probably the most common medical exam, another common procedure patients undergo is the Computerized Axial Tomography (CAT) Scan. Although the term "CAT scan" was first used, it is now commonly referred to as a CT scan. The CT scan is a very important x-ray exam that takes cross-sectional (横断的, おうだんてき) pictures of a patient's body. Common areas that CT scans are performed on are the brain, neck, and spine, as well as the chest, abdomen, and pelvic areas. The invention of the CAT scanner changed medicine forever, and was so important that the two inventors won the Nobel Prize in Physiology or Medicine in 1979.

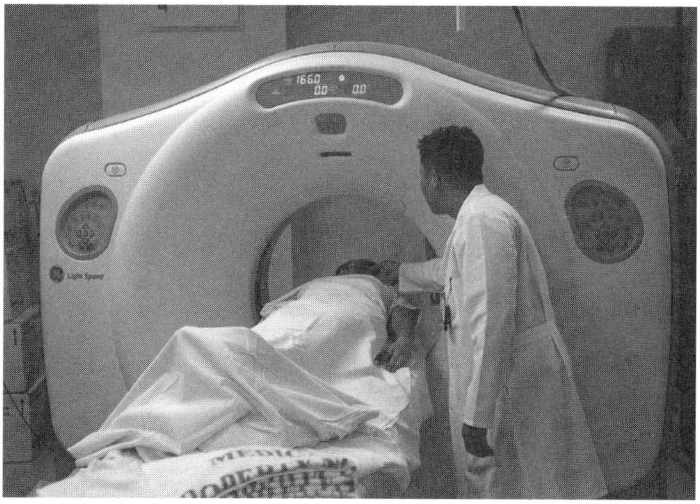

Doctors and nurses also use many other screening exams to check for potential health issues or diseases in their patients. One common test that is ordered is phlebotomy, also known as drawing blood. One reason medical professionals order blood tests is to check what's in the blood. One type of blood test measures cholesterol, commonly referred to as "good" cholesterol (high-density lipoproteins, or

HDL) and "bad" cholesterol (low-density lipoproteins, or LDL) . There are so many things that can be discovered through the blood, such as prostate specific antigen (PSA) levels and Sexually Transmitted Infections (STIs) .

Other important exams include mammograms for women and prostate exams for men. Mammograms are x-rays taken of a woman's breasts in order to check for breast cancer. Prostate exams usually involve a Digital Rectal Exam (DRE) and the PSA blood test mentioned above.

While some of these medical tests and exams may not be pleasant for some patients, they exist to help patients stay healthy and live longer lives.

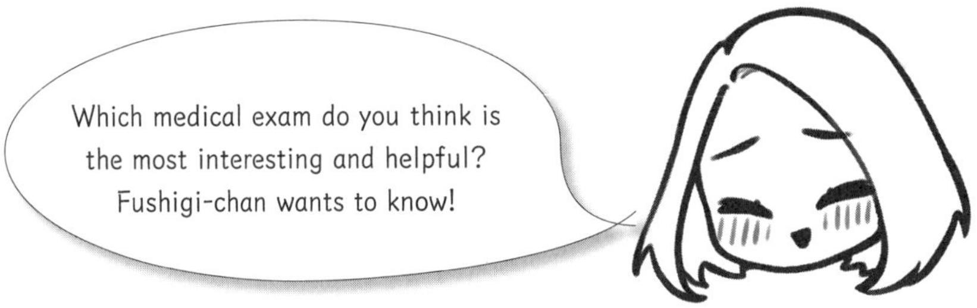

• Reading Activity 1

Answer these questions about exams.

1. How did the CT scan revolutionize the field of medicine?

2. What are two types of tests done by drawing and examining blood?

3. What is the difference between "good" and "bad" cholesterol?

4. Why is it important for women to get regularly scheduled mammograms?

5. What is the difference between the Digital Rectal Exam and the prostate specific antigen test?

• **Reading Activity 2**

Circle (T) if the statement is true or (F) if the statement is false.

1. Women have prostate glands and need prostate exams. (T・F)
2. Low-density lipoproteins are considered "bad" cholesterol. (T・F)
3. Inventors of the CAT scan received the Nobel Peace Prize in 1979. (T・F)
4. Drawing blood is known as phlebotomy. (T・F)
5. Mammograms are x-rays taken of women's breasts. (T・F)

Writing Activity

Describe two types of medical exams. What body parts are involved? What happens during the exam? What are medical professionals looking for in these tests? Write 4 or 5 sentences in the box below.

When you're finished, share your writing with a partner or the class.

Listening Activity

Listen to five people talk about medical issues they are experiencing. Which exam or procedure would you give them? Choose from the exams and procedures in the box below.

chest x-ray	pelvic exam	mammogram
physical exam	prostate exam	

Speaker 1: ______________________

Speaker 2: ______________________

Speaker 3: ______________________

Speaker 4: ______________________

Speaker 5: ______________________

Speaking Activity

In **Unit 2**, we looked at working at hospitals and clinics, and in **Unit 5**, we looked at taking medical histories. When you are working at a hospital or clinic, someone—usually an administrative staff member, but sometimes a nurse or a doctor—asks the patient to fill out a registration form. The registration form is similar to the medical history form, but much more general. Practice asking and answering questions with a partner in order to fill out the form.

Student 1: You are the doctor (nurse or administrator) , so be sure to ask polite questions to make your "patient" feel comfortable. After completing the registration form, explain to the patient which department you refer them to.

Student 2: You are the patient. When you are answering the questions, create interesting information to tell your partner! For example, change your name and nationality, think of an interesting job you have, and create a medical issue that will help your partner match you with the best department.

OUTPATIENT REGISTRATION FORM

Date	Year / Month / Day
Name	First Name Last Name
Sex	
DOB	
Age	
Nationality	
Address (city only)	
Phone #	
Occupation	
Name of Employer	
Insurance	
Current Medical Issue (explain in detail)	
Which Department to Send Patient?	( ) Internal Medicine ( ) Pediatrics ( ) ENT ( ) Obstetrics & Gynecology ( ) Neurosurgery ( ) Dermatology ( ) Psychiatry ( ) Physical Therapy ( ) Ophthalmology ( ) Orthopedics ( ) ER ( ) Other:________________

After you finish, switch roles, and complete your partner's Registration Form. When you're finished, discuss which part was most difficult to ask. Which was the most difficult to answer?

Discussion Questions

1. What are some medical exams that you have experienced? Describe them—the purpose, tools used, how the exam was performed, and, if you're comfortable, the results of the exams. How did you feel during the exams—relaxed, nervous, scared?

2. Do you believe people get enough medical exams regularly? For example, physical exams should be conducted every year, but do many people actually do them? Think

about the other exams you studied in this unit (mammograms, prostate exams, etc.) .

3. What do you know about blood? Work with a partner and list ten (10) things you know about blood. Describe each one in as much detail as possible.

Speaking Strategies: Debate Skills, Part I

In the previous unit, you learned about the reasons why debate skills are useful, as well as one standard way to hold a debate. In this unit, we'll focus on a few specific skills you should keep in mind while debating.

Final Unit Assignment

Topic Changed Perspectives

Describe your last visit to your doctor or the last medical exam you experienced (for example, the yearly physical exam from your school) . How did you feel before, during, and after the event? Did being a medical student change the way you viewed how the exam was conducted and the way the doctor or nurse presented himself/herself?

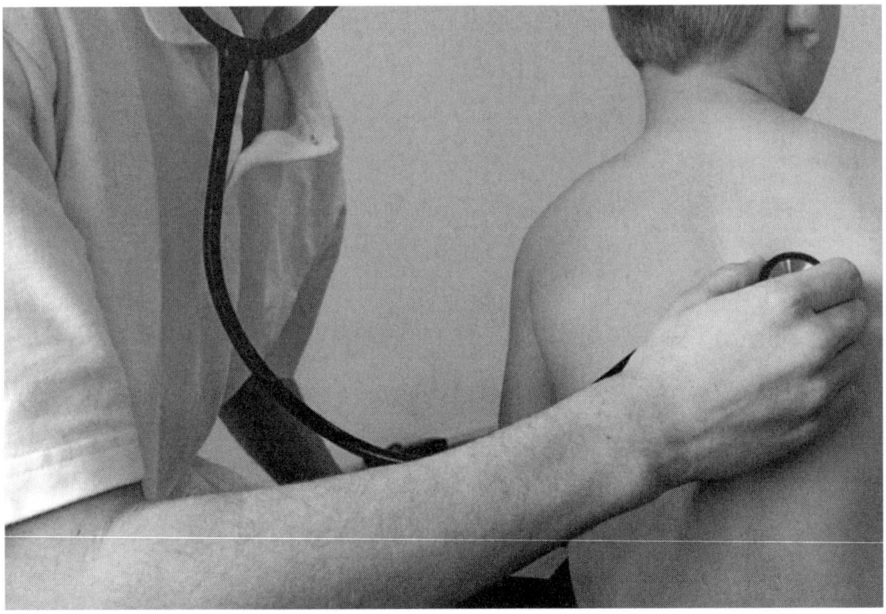

UNIT
8 Pregnancy

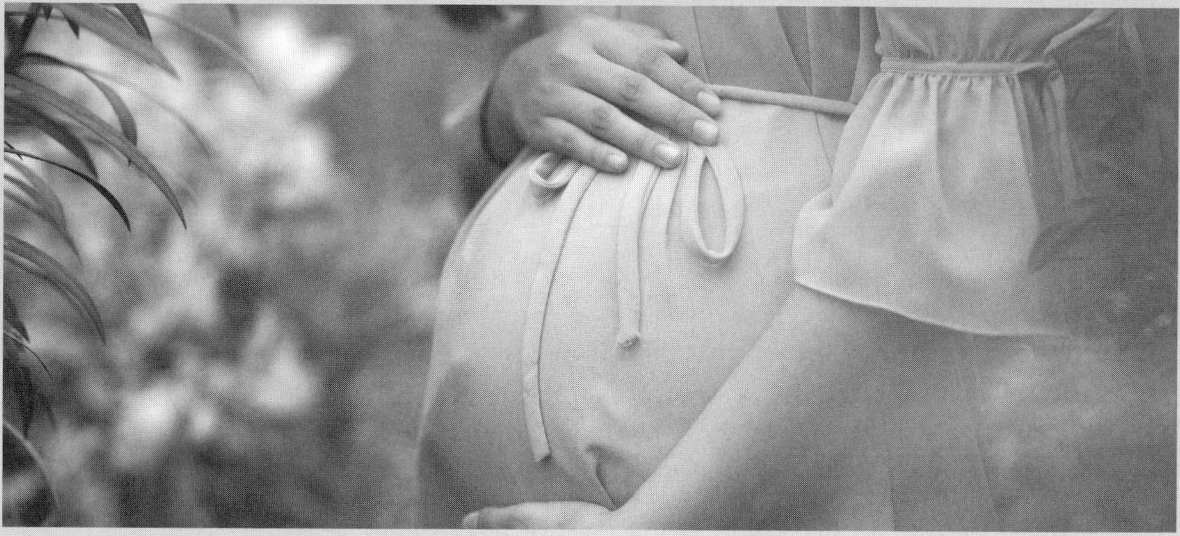

Medical Terms and Expressions

1. gynecology	婦人科 (ふじんか)
2. menstruation	生理 (せいり)
3. obstetrics	産科 (さんか)
4. midwife	助産師 (じょさんし)
5. ovulation	排卵 (はいらん)
6. pregnancy	妊娠 (にんしん)
7. labor	陣痛 (じんつう)
8. birth	誕生 (たんじょう)
9. Relax.	力を抜いてください．(ちからをぬいてください．)
10. Don't move.	動かないでください．(うごかないでください．)
11. Inhale.	息を吸ってください．(いきをすってください．)
12. Hold your breath.	息を止めてください．(いきをとめてください．)
13. Exhale.	息を吐いて下さい．(いきをはいてください．)
14. Breathe deeply.	深く息を吸ってください．(ふかくいきをすってください．)
15. Open your mouth.	口を開けてください．(くちをあけてください．)
16. Stick out your tongue.	舌を出してください．(したをだしてください．)

17. Put this under your tongue.	これを舌の下に入れてください．(これをしたのしたにいれてください．)
18. Say "ah."	「あー」と言(い)ってください．
19. Gargle with this.	これでうがいをしてください．
20. Blow into this tube.	この管に息を吐いてください．(このくだにいきをはいてください．)
21. Raise your arm.	腕を上げてください．(うでをあげてください．)
22. Raise your leg.	脚を上げてください．(あしをあげてください．)
23. Bend your elbow.	肘を曲げてください．(ひじをまげてください．)
24. Bend your knee.	膝を曲げてください．(ひざをまげてください．)
25. Bend your wrist.	手首を曲げてください．(てくびをまげてください．)
26. Roll up your sleeve.	袖をまくってください．(そでをまくってください．)
27. Make a fist.	拳を作ってください．(こぶしをつくってください．)
28. Cover your left/right eye.	右 / 左目を覆ってください．(みぎ / ひだりめをおおってください．)
29. Look at the chart.	表をご覧ください．(ひょうをごらんください．)
30. Follow my pen/finger.	ペン / 指を追ってください．(ペン / ゆびをおってください．)

31.	Take off your shoes.	靴を脱いでください．（くつをぬいでください．）
32.	Sit on the examination table.	診察台の上に座ってください．（しんさつだいのうえにすわってください．）
33.	Lie on your back (supine) .	仰向けに寝てください．（あおむけにねてください．）
34.	Lie on your side.	横向きに寝てください．（よこむきにねてください．）
35.	Lie on your stomach (prone).	うつぶせに寝てください．（うつぶせにねてください．）
36.	Put this gown on.	こちらの患者衣を着てください（こちらのかんじゃいをきてください．）
37.	Take off your shirt.	シャツを脱いでください（しゃつをぬいでください．）
38.	Pull down your pants.	ズボンを下ろしてください．（ずぼんをおろしてください．）
39.	Take off your clothes.	衣服を脱いでください．（いふくをぬいでください．）
40.	Don't bathe for 24 hours.	24時間はシャワーを浴びたり，お風呂に入らないでください．（24じかんはしゃわーをあびたり，おふろにはいらないでください．）

Medical Expressions: Practice

Without looking at the list above, write the English translation for the following Japanese phrases.

1) 肘を曲げてください．

2) 息を吐いて下さい．

3)「あー」と言ってください．

4) 袖をまくってください．

5) 動かないでください．

6) 衣服を脱いでください．

7) 深く息をしてください．

8) 口を開けてください．

9) 膝を曲げてください．

10) 診察台の上に座ってください．

Grammar Review: Roots

In the past two units, you learned about prefixes—letters at the beginning of words—and suffixes—letters at the end of words. Root words, like the roots of a tree, are the foundation of words. Root words have no prefixes or suffixes, and are the basic part of words.

Many root words can be traced back to Greek or Latin, and usually do not form a complete word on their own (although there are root words that do form a complete word, such as *act* and *norm*) .

Here are ten root words and how they change their meanings with the addition of prefixes and suffixes.

Root word	Meaning	With prefix or suffix + meaning
act	do something	**action**: The process of doing something, usually to achieve a goal
norm	usual, typical	**normal**: usual, typical or expected
corp	body	**corpse**: a dead body
cred	believe	**incredible**: hard to believe
gen	birth	**genetics**: related to heredity or genes
micro	small	**microscope**: tool used to view very small objects
multi	many	**multilingual**: a person who speaks many languages
sect	cut apart	**dissect**: cut up in order to study the internal parts
sen	old	**senior**: older or higher ranking person
tele	far	**telephone**: a phone

Although many of the words above are related to medicine, here are ten common root words found specifically in medical terms.

Root word	Meaning	Example word / 日本語
abdomin/o	abdomen	abdominal cavity / 腹腔 (ふくくう)
arteri/o	artery	arteriogram / 動脈図 (どうみゃくず)
bronch/i/o	bronchus	bronchitis / 気管支炎 (きかんしえん)
col/o	colon	colorectal cancer / 大腸がん (だいちょうがん)
derm/a/o	skin	dermatitis / 皮膚炎 (ひふえん)
gynec/o	female	gynecology / 婦人科学 (ふじんかがく)
hemat/o	blood	hematologis / 血液学者 (けつえきがくしゃ)
my/o	muscle	myalgia / 筋肉痛 (きんにくつう)
path/o	disease	pathology / 病理学 (びょうりがく)
thorac/o	chest	thoracic aorta / 胸部大動脈 (きょうぶだいどうみゃく)

These twenty root words are just a small part of a very large group, so, as mentioned in previous units, you should study a medical terminology book in order to get a complete understanding of the roots, as well as the prefixes and suffixes, that make up medical terminology. Remember that if you can understand even one of the three parts of a word, you have a good chance of understanding the general meaning of many medical words.

• Grammar Activity 1

Circle the best answer for each question or statement. You may need to use a medical dictionary to help with some of the answers.

1. Which one is the plural form of *thorax*?

   [a. thoracos b. thoraces c. thoraxis d. thoracic]

2. Which suffix cannot be used with the root *hemato*?

   [a. -logy b. -cele c. -gen d. -ist]

3. Which of the following is not a root word?

   [a. leukocyte b. laparo c. pharmac d. gastro]

4. What does the root *ophthalm* mean?

   [a. nerve b. eyes c. sight d. lungs]

5. Choose the correct suffix to add to the root word *sept* to make it mean "relating to sepsis, or a systemic infection."

   [a. -ic b. -is c. -oscopy d. -al]

• Grammar Activity 2

Use the example root words or phrases in the **Grammar Review** section to complete the sentences.

1. My GP referred me to a ________________ because she thinks I might be anemic.

2. According to the CDC ________________ ________________ is the fourth most common cancer among men and women.

3. ________________ , or inflammation of the skin, is usually characterized by itchy red

skin.

4. The ________ ________ is a continuation of the descending aorta, and is located in the thorax.

5. If you're interested in helping women with medical issues, especially diseases of the reproductive organs, you should consider becoming a ________ .

• Grammar Activity 3

Match the root words with a suffix to make a medical term. After you choose the suffix, write the entire word below and then check the meaning in a medical English dictionary.

1. carcino •	• a. plasm
2. cyto •	• b. flexion
3. laparo •	• c. genic
4. dorsi •	• d. graphy
5. adeno •	• e. scopy

word		meaning
1. ________	:	________
2. ________	:	________
3. ________	:	________
4. ________	:	________
5. ________	:	________

Reading with Fushigi-chan: Pregnancy Stories

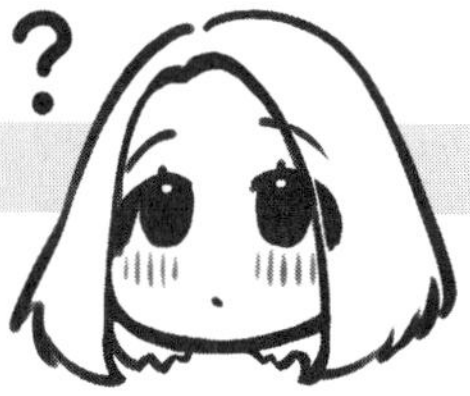

Pregnancy is both an amazing and mysterious part of life. So many complex systems in the body work together to make conception (in other words, getting pregnant), pregnancy (usually lasting nine months, or three trimesters) , and birth possible. Although sometimes a situation can occur that makes childbirth difficult or impossible for some women, pregnancy is a process that usually ends with a crying baby, a happy mother, and a relieved family. There are many amazing facts that provide a better insight into what pregnancy and childbirth mean to expecting mothers.

For example, the longest time a woman went carrying her unborn baby inside her was 375 days. Mrs. Beulah Hunter was 25 years old when she was pregnant, but didn't give birth for 375 days, which is about 100 days longer than normal pregnancies. (Source: Time, 1945)

Compared to the longest pregnancy ever, the shortest birth was an unbelievable 21 weeks and 4 days, making the baby the earliest premature baby to survive the birthing process. There were some complications, as would be expected, but the baby ended up surviving, and is now a happy and healthy child with no physical or mental disabilities. (Source: USA Today, 2017)

According to Guinness World Records, the oldest woman to ever give birth was 66-year-old Maria del Carmen Bousada Lara. Born in Spain, she gave birth to twin boys by caesarean section (commonly referred to as a C-section) on December 29, 2006. One interesting point about this story is that Maria was rejected for in vitro fertilization (IVF) treatment in Spain because of her age, so she went to America and lied about her age. After they believed she was 55 years old, she received IVF treatment and became pregnant. (Source: Guinness World Records, 2022)

The most babies a woman has ever successfully given birth to was eight! In 2006, Nadya Suleman gave birth to 6 boys and 2 girls, all conceived via IVF treatment. Famously known as "Octomom" because eight children born at the same time are referred to as octuplets, Ms. Suleman became a celebrity due to the heavy media coverage of her unusual pregnancy. (Source: Guinness World Records, 2021)

These are just some of the interesting, unusual, and amazing stories related to pregnancy.

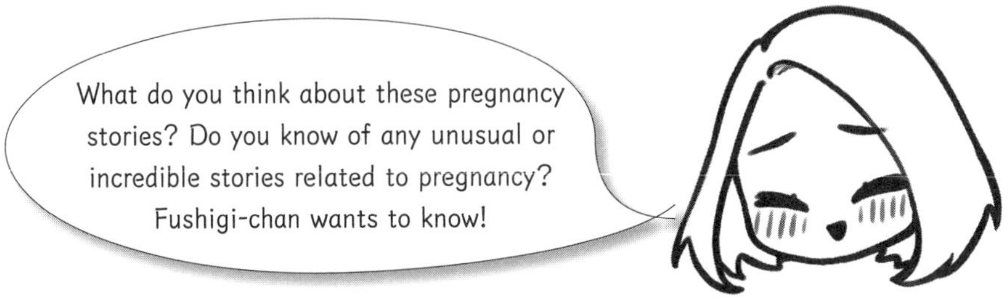

• Reading Activity 1

Circle (T) if the statement is true or (F) if the statement is false.

1. Eight babies born at the same time are called octomom. (T・F)
2. Maria lied about her age in order to get IVF in Spain. (T・F)
3. A typical pregnancy usually lasts about 9 months. (T・F)
4. The shortest birth was twenty-one weeks and four days. (T・F)
5. Beulah Hunter had a normal pregnancy with no complications. (T・F)

• Reading Activity 2

Fill in the blanks with the appropriate words.

1. *In vitro fertilization* is often shortened to ________________ .
2. Nadya Suleman gave birth to ________________ boys and ________________ girls, and became known as ________________ .
3. The earliest premature baby survived and had no ________________ or ________________ disabilities.
4. A *C-section* is also known as a ________________ ________________ .
5. Beulah Hunter was ________________ years old when she was pregnant, but didn't give birth for ________________ days, which is ________________ days longer than normal pregnancies.

Writing Activity

In what ways would you support a worried patient who comes to you after finding out she's pregnant? What questions would you ask her to better understand her situation? Write 4 or 5 questions in the box provided.

When you're finished, share your questions with a partner or the class!

Listening Activity

Listen to two women talk about their experiences with their doctors and nurses during pregnancy. What are the positive points that they share? What could the doctors and nurses have done better to support them?

Speaker 1

Name:____________________

Positive points:____

____

____

Areas to improve:____

____

____

Speaker 2

Name: ____________________

Positive points: ____

____

____

Areas to improve: ____

____

____

Speaking Activity

Checking information is important in the medical field. One small error could cause a misunderstanding between doctors, nurses or wards that could lead to a medical incident, such as prescribing the wrong medication or dosage. In this activity, you are going to confirm information about a patient.

Two women were just admitted to the hospital with pregnancy complications. Confirm the women's information with a partner.

Student A: Use the form on the next page. Do not show your partner. Your form has the patient's correct information (name, birthdate, etc.) . When your partner, Student B, asks to confirm the information, make sure you give him or her the correct information by speaking slowly and clearly. After you give the information, ask your partner to repeat the information back to you.

Student B: Use the form that is at the end of this unit. Do not show your partner. You need to confirm the patient's information and correct the mistakes. Remember to ask, "Is this correct?" If you don't hear your partner clearly, say, "Pardon?" or "I'm sorry, could you repeat that?" Double-check what you wrote down to ensure it is correct.

Student A
Surname: Suzuki
First name: Runa
Sex: F
Marital Status: Single
Address: 12-7-3 Osaka Sky Tree
Phone: 040-749-32217
Occupation: massage therapist
GP: Dr. Green
PC: abdominal pain
Notes: 5 months pregnant

Discussion Questions

1. Describe sex education in the country you were raised. When does it start, or does it occur at all? What could be done to improve young men and women's perspectives on relationships, sex, abstinence (禁欲, きんよく), and pregnancy.
2. Are pregnant women supported enough in your country? Do men have access to resources, as well?
3. How are births celebrated amongst family members and friends? Are there special rituals, traditions, and holidays to celebrate new births and children in general?

Speaking Strategies: Casual Speech versus Formal Speech

"Hey, what's up?"

"How are you doing today?"

Most people can probably identify which question above is the casual one. However, with the popularity of social media sites and blogs, casual speech is becoming more and more acceptable in formal settings. Even politicians and company CEOs have opted for a more casual tone in order to connect with the "average" customer or voter. It is important, therefore, to understand the different levels of not only English, but any language you speak. Whether you are fluent or just learning "survival language" skills for travel, it is best to know when to say what to whom. Casual language has the power to not only make you sound fluent, but it can make also help you make friends with local people, learn new idiomatic expressions and slang words, and blend into the culture more easily.

Final Unit Assignment

Topic What's up, doc?

What are some pros and cons of using casual speech in medical situations? Think of three advantages and three disadvantages, and give examples for each point you make. When would it be most appropriate to use casual speech in a medical situation?

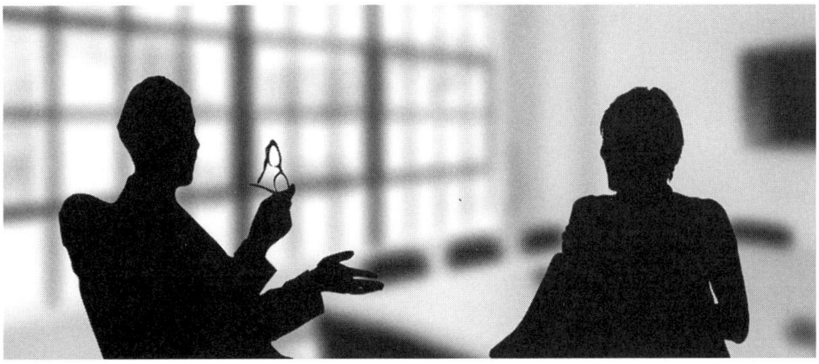

Speaking Activity: Student B

Student B: Use the form below. Do not show your partner. You need to confirm the patient's information and correct the mistakes. Remember to ask, "Is this correct?" If you don't hear your partner clearly, say, "Pardon?" or "I'm sorry, could you repeat that?" Double-check what you wrote down to ensure it is correct..

Student B
Surname: Sasaki
First name: Rina
Sex: F
Marital Status: Widowed
Address: 1-17-30 Tokyo Sky Tree
Phone: 090-742-08227
Occupation: physical therapist
GP: Dr. Greenwich
PC: internal bleeding
Notes: 8 months pregnant

UNIT 9

Cancer, Part 1

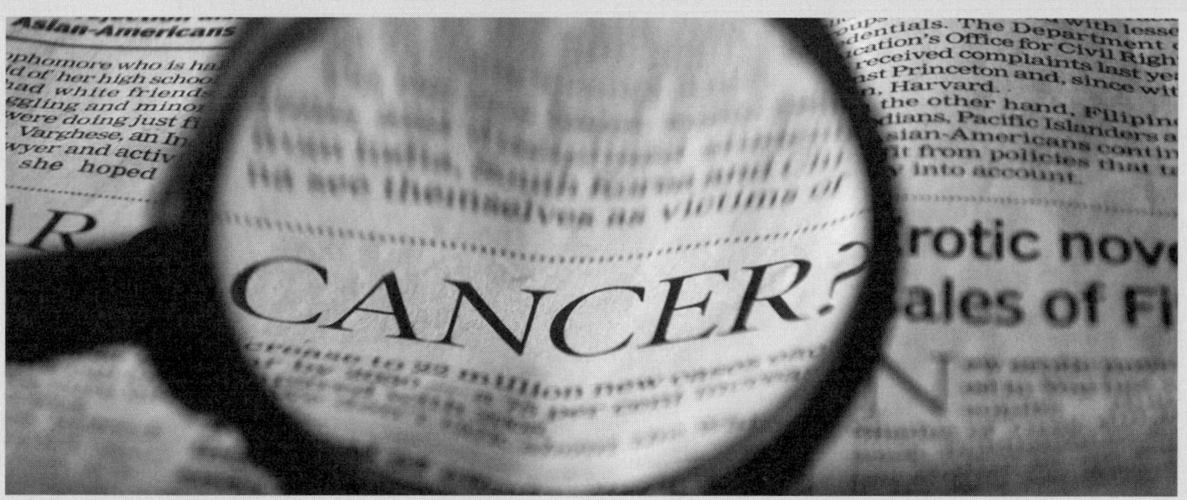

Medical Terms

1. scratch	引っ掻き傷（ひっかききず）
2. cut	切り傷（きりきず）
3. bruise	打ち身（うちみ）， 打撲傷（だぼくしょう）
4. fracture	骨折（こっせつ）
5. scar	傷跡（きずあと）
6. cold	風邪（かぜ）
7. influenza	流行性感冒（りゅうこうせいかんぼう）
8. pneumonia	肺炎（はいえん）
9. bronchitis	気管支炎（きかんしえん）
10. asthma	喘息（ぜんそく）
11. blood clot	血栓（けっせん）
12. arteriosclerosis	動脈硬化症（どうみゃくこうかしょう）
13. cancer (lung, stomach, rectal)	がん（肺，胃，直腸）
14. leukemia	白血病（はっけつびょう）
15. angina pectoris	狭心症（きょうしんしょう）
16. myocardial infarction	心筋梗塞（しんきんこうそく）
17. tuberculosis	結核（けっかく）
18. cerebral hemorrhage	脳出血（のうしゅっけつ）
19. aneurysm	動脈瘤（どうみゃくりゅう）
20. anemia	貧血（ひんけつ）

21. appendicitis	虫垂炎（ちゅうすいえん）
22. ulcer	潰瘍（かいよう）
23. liver cirrhosis	肝硬変（かんこうへん）
24. hernia	ヘルニア
25. nephritis	腎炎（じんえん）
26. enlarged prostate	前立腺肥大症（ぜんりつせんひだいしょう）
27. cystitis	膀胱炎（ぼうこうえん）
28. hepatitis (A, B, C)	（A, B, C 型［がた］）肝炎（かんえん）
29. syphilis	梅毒（ばいどく）
30. gonorrhea	淋病（りんびょう）
31. chlamydia	クラミジア
32. sexually transmitted infection	性感染症（せいかんせんしょう）
33. kidney stone	腎臓結石（じんぞうけっせき）
34. breast cancer	乳（にゅう）がん
35. uterine cancer	子宮（しきゅう）がん
36. deaf	聾（ろう）
37. blind	盲（もう），失明（しつめい）， 視覚消失（しかくしょうしつ）
38. mute	聴唖（ちょうあ）
39. arthritis	関節炎（かんせつえん）
40. menopause	更年期（こうねんき）

Medical Terms: Practice

Match the medical terms (1-10) to their Japanese translation (a-j).

1) uterine cancer	•	•	a. 腎臓結石（じんぞうけっせき）
2) syphilis	•	•	b. 子宮（しきゅう）がん
3) anemia	•	•	c. 切り傷（きりきず）
4) asthma	•	•	d. 脳出血（のうしゅっけつ）
5) appendicitis	•	•	e. 結核（けっかく）
6) kidney stone	•	•	f. 梅毒（ばいどく）
7) deaf	•	•	g. 貧血（ひんけつ）
8) tuberculosis	•	•	h. 喘息（ぜんそく）
9) cerebral hemorrhage	•	•	i. 虫垂炎（ちゅうすいえん）
10) cut	•	•	j. 聾（ろう）

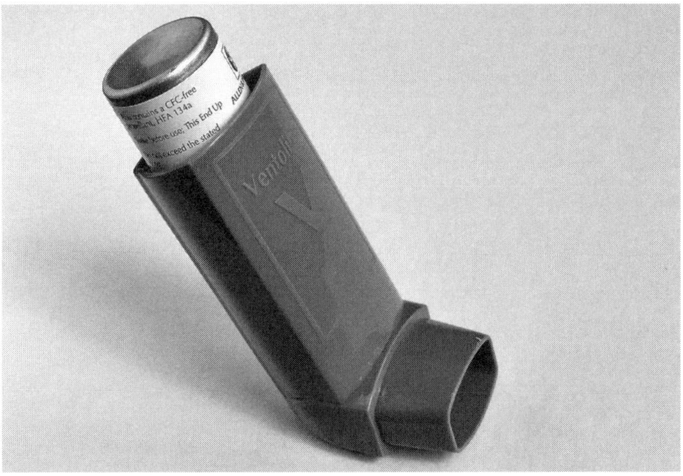

Grammar Review: Countable and Uncountable Nouns

We learned in a previous chapter that nouns are people, places, and things. There are certain nouns that you can count. For example, *nurses* (people) , *hospitals* (places) , and *syringes* (things) can all be counted. These types of nouns are called **Countable Nouns**.

The hospital recently hired twelve nurses for the ICU.
Please place four syringes in the silver tray.

There are some nouns that cannot be counted. For example, *oxygen*, *fluid*, and *steam* are all uncountable—you cannot count them unless they are in some kind of sack or container. These types of nouns are called **Uncountable Nouns** (also called **Noncount Nouns**) .

How much oxygen is left?
Is the patient getting enough fluids?

When using countable and uncountable nouns, we can use words like *some*, *much*, *many*, and *any* to talk about quantity (how many) .

Countable nouns

There are many **doctors** in the operating room.

Are there any **syringes** left?

Uncountable nouns

The hospital cafeteria ran out of **rice**!

How much **medicine** should I give to the patient? (Note: *medicine* can be a countable and uncountable noun)

• Grammar Activity 1

Look at the words in the box and decide if they are countable or uncountable nouns (or both) . Put them in the correct column.

disease	health	water	pills
bread	clinic	scrubs	

uncountable	countable

• Grammar Activity 2

Read the questions below. Write *a* or *an* before countable nouns, and a dash (—) before uncountable nouns.

1. Do you think it's a good idea to pour ______ salt on a wound?
2. Are you interested in working at ______ women's clinic?
3. Do you usually have ______ sandwich for lunch?
4. How much ______ red wine would you recommend your patients to drink?
5. Is ordering ______ glass of red wine with dinner an unhealthy choice?
6. Some surgeons listen to ______ music while they operate. Is this safe?
7. Do patients need to be careful of ______ mercury levels in tuna?
8. How much ______ furniture will you put in your office?
9. Do you get enough ______ sleep?
10. Do you want to work at ______ big hospital when you finish medical school?

• Grammar Activity 3

Ask your partner the questions in **Activity 2** and write down their answers below.

My partner's name: ____________________

His/Her answers:

1. ____
2. ____
3. ____
4. ____

5. ______________________________

6. ______________________________

7. ______________________________

8. ______________________________

9. ______________________________

10. ______________________________

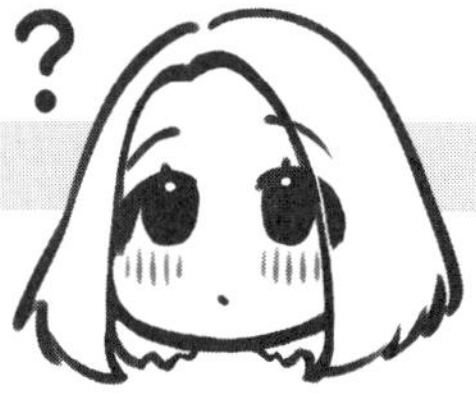

Reading with Fushigi-chan: Cancers

Cancer is never an easy topic to talk about, but it's an important one, especially for doctors, nurses, and other medical professionals. In medicine, a lot of focus is given to cancers, and rightly so. The more knowledgeable medical professionals are about the various types of cancers and treatments, the better they can support and protect their patients' health.

Cancer is one of the main causes of death worldwide, and nearly 10 million people died from cancer in 2020 (Ferlay, et al., 2020) . According to the World Health Organization (2020) , here are the most common forms of cancer, along with the number of cases:

- breast cancer (2.26 million cases) ;
- lung cancer (2.21 million cases) ;
- colon and rectal cancer (1.93 million cases) ;
- prostate cancer (1.41 million cases) ;
- skin cancer (1.20 million cases) ; and
- stomach cancer (1.09 million cases) .

The most common causes of cancer deaths were:

- lung cancer (1.80 million deaths) ;
- colon and rectal cancer (916,000 deaths) ;
- liver cancer (830,000 deaths) ;
- stomach cancer (769,000 deaths) ; and
- breast cancer (685,000 deaths) .

To make matters more difficult, there are many things can cause cancer. There are some that people simply cannot avoid, like the sun or contaminants in food and water. Infections from viruses and bacteria can also cause cancer. However, there are some things that cause cancer that can be avoided, such as drinking alcohol, smoking cigarettes, and eating carcinogenic foods like processed meats and fried foods.

Although smoking cigarettes, drinking alcohol, eating unhealthy food, and not exercising are all choices that people make, these are choices that can be changed. By making the right choices, people can become healthier, stronger, and fitter, making their body better prepared to fight cancer cells. According to WHO (2020) , "Between 30 and 50% of cancers can currently be prevented by avoiding risk factors and implementing existing evidence-based prevention strategies." Also, many cancers can be treated when detected early, so screening tests are vital in the fight against cancer.

Hopefully there will be a cure for cancer one day, but until then medical professionals should do their best to promote prevention strategies.

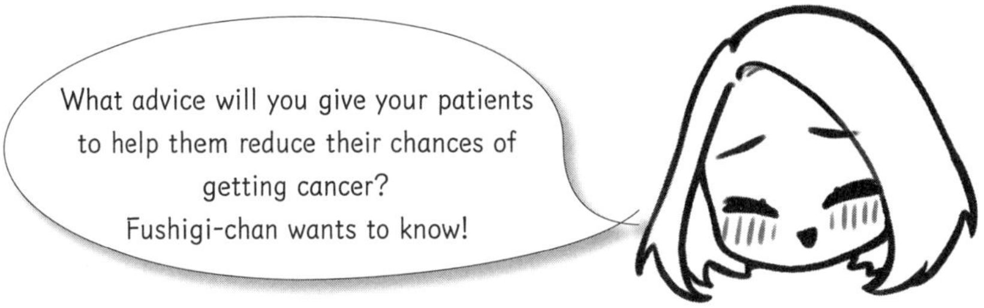

• Reading Activity 1

Answer these questions about cancer.

1. Why is it difficult to control the number of cancer cases?

2. What are some ways people can reduce their risk of getting cancer?

3. What is the difference between colon and rectal cancer?

4. How can people protect themselves from harmful sun rays?

5. Why do you think breast and lung cancer are so prevalent (流行る, はやる)?

____

____

• Reading Activity 2

Fill in the blanks with the missing words.

1. The more ____________ doctors and nurses are about cancer, the better they can treat their patients.

2. According to WHO, the most common form of cancer is ____________ cancer.

3. There are some things that cause cancer that people stop doing, such as ____________ and ____________ ____________ .

4. Between ________ and ________ % of cancers can currently be prevented.

5. ____________ ____________ are really important because many cancers can be treated when detected early.

Writing Activity

What are some reasons people continue to smoke, drink, eat junk food, and not exercise? What are some ways you can convince them to change unhealthy habits? Write 4-5 sentences in the box below.

When you're finished, share your writing with a partner or the class.

Listening Activity

Listen to a person talk about why he continues to smoke tobacco even though there is a risk of getting cancer. While you're listening, fill in the missing information in the excerpts below.

Speaker's Name: ____________________

First, smoking has become a habit that is hard to break. I have been smoking for about ____________ years, so lighting up a cigarette is almost second nature to me. Over the years, smoking has become such a big part of my daily ________________ that going without a cigarette feels ________________ And I'm scared that kicking this habit will require a tremendous amount of ________________ .

Second, smoking helps reduce my ________________ and ________________ . Whenever I'm feeling stressed out at work or in my personal life, a cigarette can help me calm down.

Finally, I simply enjoy the ________________ of smoking. However, I understand that the long-term health ________________ are simply not worth it even though smoking may be enjoyable in the moment.

Speaking Activity: Giving Advice

When someone gives advice to another person, it is important to soften their words so that they don't hurt their feelings. Also, it is important to encourage them to consider their suggestions. There are phrases that can be used when giving advice.

You should try...	Maybe you can try...
You should consider...	Have you thought about...
You could...	I suggest...
My advice would be...	I recommend...
Why don't you...	If I were you, ...

Work with a partner and give each other advice about the situations below. Practice each scenario, with one student expressing the problem ("I can't stop smoking! What should I do?") and the other student giving advice ("Maybe you can first try switching to e-cigarettes.") . Be sure to respond to the advice in some way ("Thanks, but I've already tried e-cigarettes." Or "That's a good idea. I never thought of that.") .

Student 1

Situation	Advice Received
"I drink too much coffee each day. I can't stop!"	
"I've gained 6 kg in the last month. What should I do?"	

Student 2

Situation	Advice Received
"I never have time to do homework. I have too many things to do."	
"I don't like going to hospitals or clinics, so I haven't gotten a physical exam in years."	

Act out the situations in front of another group or the entire class. Afterwards, discuss how the advice could have been improved in order to encourage the person to change their habits and routines.

Discussion Questions

1. Is there enough information and resources about cancer, or do you think more should be done to make people aware of cancer dangers?
2. Do you think a cure for cancer will ever be found? Why or why not? When do you predict a cure will be found?
3. Is it realistic (or even possible) to ban cigarettes, alcohol, and junk food if it means the global community will be healthier and live longer? How would you go about banning them?

Speaking Strategies: Formal Speech versus Casual Speech

In the previous unit, we looked at casual speech, which can include jargon, idiomatic expressions, slang, and even offensive language ("curse words") . Casual speech is an important part of any language and can give the speaker a sense of fluency that may lead to better understanding of the culture and closer friendships. That said, formal speech is by far the best way to speak a language for several reasons. The most important, though, is that formal speech is almost always well received by the listeners. Most conversations spoken with formal speech, which includes polite, respectful language, will be taken in positive ways. Whether you're talking to a teacher, a police officer, a convenience store employee or a stranger, formal speech should always be used.

Final Unit Assignment

Topic A cure for cancer, but...

Your medical team has discovered a cure for cancer! However, there are only enough materials to cure 1,000,000 (1 million) people.

How will your team decide who gets the cure? What is your **rationale**（論法, ろんぽう ; reasons for doing something）for choosing them? How will you share your discovery and limitations to the general public? How will you prepare for any **backlash**（反発, はんぱつ, バックラッシュ ; angry responses）?

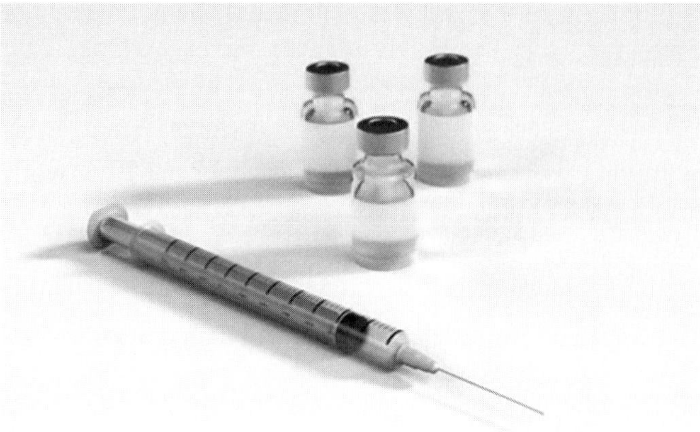

UNIT

10 Cancer, Part 2

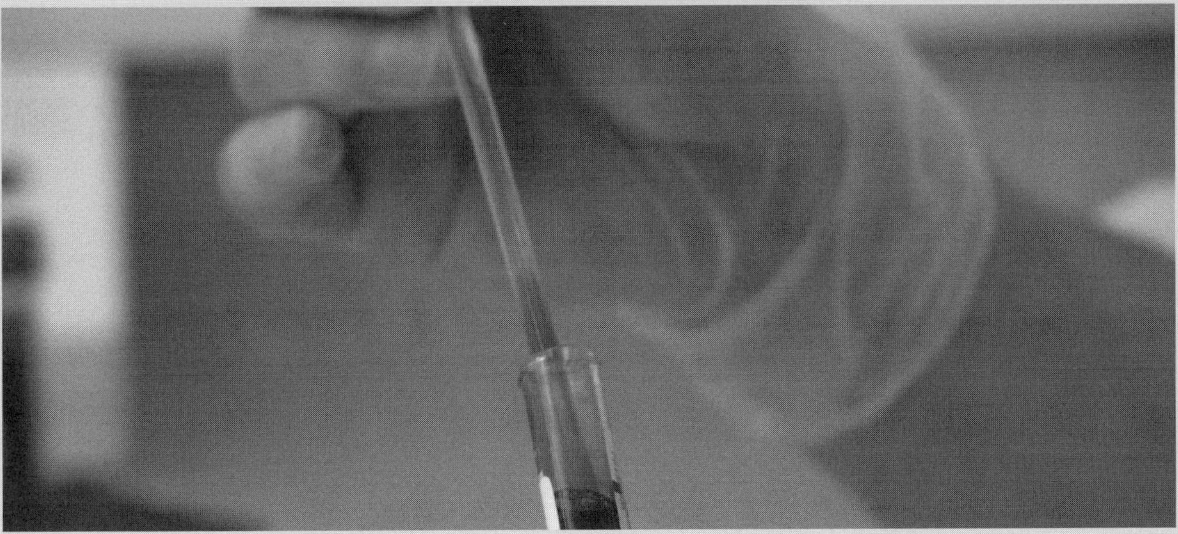

Medical Terms and Expressions

1. oncology	腫瘍学 (しゅようがく)
2. radiology	放射線科 (ほうしゃせんか)
3. urology	泌尿器科 (ひにょうきか)
4. hematology	血液学 (けつえきがく)
5. Take this medicine once a day.	こちらのお薬は1日に1回飲んでください．(こちらのおくすりはいちにちにいっかいのんでください．)
6. Take this medicine before meals.	こちらのお薬は食前に飲んでください．(こちらのおくすりはしょくぜんにのんでください．)
7. Take this before bedtime.	こちらは寝る前に飲んでください．(こちらはねるまえにのんでください．)
8. Don't drive after taking this.	飲んだ後は運転はしないでください．(のんだあとはうんてんをひかえてください．)
9. Fill this cup with urine.	こちらのコップに尿を入れてください．(こちらのこっぷににょうをいれてください．)
10. Rest for the next 24 hours.	24時間は安静にしていてください．(24じかんはあんせいにしていてください．)
11. Follow this diet.	この通りに食事をとってください．(このとおりにしょくじをとってください．)
12. Go to the ______ department.	____科へお問い合わせください．(____かへおといあわせください．)

13. medical expenses	医療費 (いりょうひ)
14. natural death	自然死 (しぜんし)
15. internal medicine	内科 (ないか)
16. general practitioner	一般開業医 (いっぱんかいぎょうい)
17. registered nurse	正看護師 (せいかんごし)
18. neurology	神経科 (しんけいか)
19. ophthalmology	眼科 (がんか)
20. otolaryngology	耳鼻咽喉科 (じびいんこうか)
21. cardiology	心臓病学 (しんぞうびょうがく)
22. gastroenterology	胃腸病科 (いちょうびょうか)
23. endocrinology	内分泌科 (ないぶんぴつか)
24. anesthesiology	麻酔科 (ますいか)
25. neurosurgery	脳神経外科 (のうしんけいげか)
26. paramedic	救急医療士(きゅうきゅういりょうし)
27. Emergency Medical Technician	救急隊員 (きゅうきゅうたいいん)
28. physical therapist	理学療法士 (りがくりょうほうし)
29. lab technician	検査技師 (けんさぎし)
30. X-ray technician	X線技師 (えっくすせんぎし)
31. MRI technician	MRI技師 (えむあーるあいぎし)

32. pharmacist	薬剤師 (やくざいし)
33. orderly	看護補助員 (かんごほじょいん)
34. orthopedics	整形外科 (せいけいげか)
35. podiatry	足病学 (そくびょうがく)
36. dentistry	歯学 (しがく)

37. plastic surgery	形成外科 (けいせいげか)
38. dermatology	皮膚科 (ひふか)
39. speech therapist	言語聴覚士 (げんごちょうかくし)
40. psychiatry	精神科 (せいしんか)

Medical Terms: Practice

Match the medical terms (1-10) to their definitions (a-j).

1) ____ oncology •　　• a. person trained to help women in childbirth

2) ____ internal medicine •　　• b. study of the physiology of blood

3) ____ paramedic •　　• c. branch of medicine dealing with skin disorders

4) ____ pediatrics •　　• d. branch of medicine dealing with elderly patients

5) ____ midwife •　　• e. branch of medicine dealing with children

6) ____ geriatrics •　　• f. doctor who provides primary healthcare to patients

7) ____ gynecology •　　• g. the study and treatment of cancer

8) ____ hematology •　　• h. branch of medicine dealing with diseases of women and girls

9) ____ general practitioner •　　• i. a person trained to give emergency medical care

10) ____ dermatology •　　• j. medical specialty dealing with the treatment of internal diseases

Grammar Review: Simple Past and Past Perfect

We use the simple past tense to talk about activities or events that happened in the past. We add -ed to the end of most verbs to form the simple past. If the verb ends in -e, then we only add -d.

The hospital opened in 1860.
The patient needed the operation as quickly as possible.

Some verbs have special spellings. These verbs are called irregular verbs because they do not use -ed or -d. For example, *be* changes to *was/were*.

Be careful not to mistake the past tense with the **past perfect tense**. The past perfect tense is also used to describe actions that started in the past and are completed, but it is used to highlight an action that happened *before* another one. The past perfect tense is formed using the auxiliary verb "had" + the past participle of a verb. For example:

Past: She spoke to the patient.
Past Perfect: She had spoken to the patient before the surgery.

As you can see from the example above and the chart below, sometimes the past participle is different from the simple past form.

Verb	Past	Past perfect
speak	spoke	spoken
go	went	gone

• Grammar Activity 1

Change these verbs to the past. Then write the Past Perfect form of the verb (write "had [past participle]").

Infinitive (辞書形)	Past	Past perfect
e.g., be	was/were	had been
do	1)	
have	2)	
can	3)	
go	4)	
make	5)	
give	6)	
take	7)	

write	8)	
think	9)	
tell	10)	

• Grammar Activity 2

Complete the dialogue with the correct form of the verb in parentheses. The past perfect and other forms can be used.

Doctor: Hello, Ms. Sakai. You ____________ (have) surgery before, correct?

Ms. Sakai: Yes, my appendix ____________ (rupture) , so I ____________ (need) it ______________ (remove) .

Doctor: _________ you _____________ (receive) medical attention before it was removed?

Ms. Sakai: I ____________ (feel) a little nauseous before that, but I don't think it was related to my appendix.

Doctor: I see. Well, we'll monitor you carefully to make sure there are no complications. ___________ (do) it difficult to talk to your husband about your decision to have surgery?

Ms. Sakai: No. He ___________ (be) very supportive before, so it was easy to talk to him about it now.

Doctor: That's good. It seems like you _____________ (make) up your mind to have surgery, but it's always good to have family support.

Ms. Sakai: I only wish I ____________ (decided) to do this years ago.

• Grammar Activity 3

Now work with a new partner and write a new dialogue similar to the one in **Activity 2**. Make sure you use verbs in the past tense. Other tenses are OK to use, too!

Student A: ____

____

Student B: ____

____

Student A: ____

____

Student B: ____

____

Student A: ____

____

Student B: ____

____

Student A: ____

____

Student B: ____

____

Reading with Fushigi-chan: Bad News

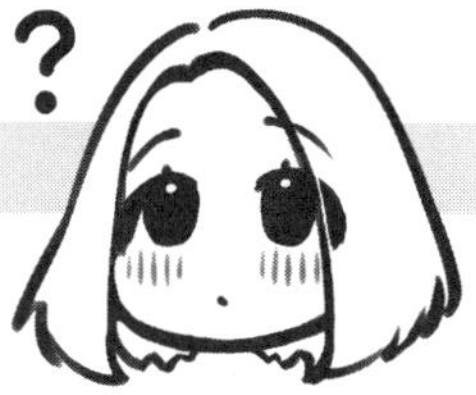

"I'm sorry, ma'am, I broke your window with a baseball."

"Please forgive me. I just ran over your cat."

"I'm so sorry. I lost the keys to your apartment."

Giving bad news is never easy to do, especially if you are admitting to something you did wrong. Imagine giving someone bad news when you played no part in the incident. When you become a medical professional, you will often have to give patients bad news about extremely difficult situations. Whether it is about a loved one who passed away (亡くなる, なくなる) or a recent discovery of cancer, as a medical professional you must be prepared to deliver this bad news to your patients with care.

Fortunately, Baile, Buckman, Lenzi, Glober, Beale, and Kudelka (2020) created SPIKES—a 6-step approach to deliver bad news to patients. It is never enjoyable to give a person bad news, especially to someone who has been suffering or wasn't expecting the news, but it is part of a medical professional's job. Therefore, doctors, nurses, and other medical professionals must practice so they can deliver the news delicately and compassionately. The six steps of SPIKES are:

S: **S**et up the interview. (Make sure it is private and includes family members, if necessary.)

P: Evaluate the patient's **P**erception. (Do they know what the medical issue is and how serious it is?)

I: Get the patient's **I**nvitation. (Do they want the information? If so, how much do they want to hear?)

K: Give **K**nowledge to the Patient. (Warn them you have bad news, and speak in layman's terms—not complex medical terminology.)

E: Address the patient's **E**motions with **E**mpathy. (This is the most difficult part because the patient may be angry, crying, silent or in denial.)

S: Have a **S**trategy and **S**ummarize. (Having a plan will help to reduce a patient's anxiety. Also, make sure the patient understands what is happening by summarizing in order to check their understanding.)

Here is an example taken from Baile, et al.'s (2020) article:

DOCTOR: I'm sorry to say that the x-ray shows that the chemotherapy doesn't seem to be working [pause] . Unfortunately, the tumor has grown somewhat.

PATIENT: I've been afraid of this! [Cries]

DOCTOR: [Moves his chair closer, offers the patient a tissue, and pauses.] I know that this isn't what you wanted to hear. I wish the news were better.

Giving bad news is never easy, and although it is a difficult situation to think about and practice, medical professionals can improve the ways they approach giving bad news so that their patients feel understood and supported.

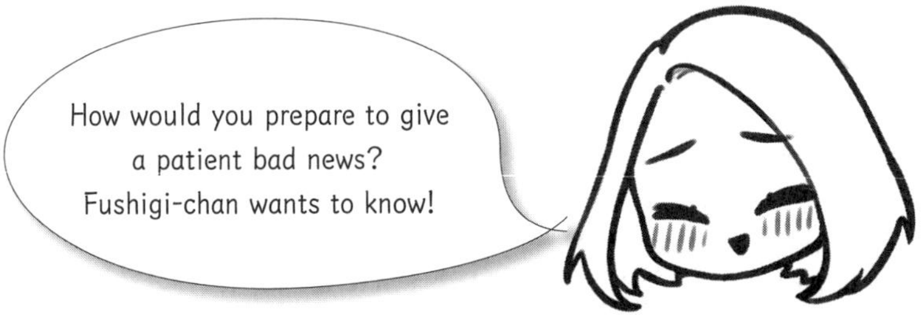

• Reading Activity 1

Circle (T) if the statement is true or (F) if the statement is false.

1. Giving bad news is not difficult. (T・F)
2. SPIKES is a 5-step approach to give a patient bad news. (T・F)
3. The patient always wants information about a bad health situation. (T・F)
4. Giving bad news is part of a medical professional's duties. (T・F)
5. Delicacy and compassion are important when giving bad news. (T・F)

• Reading Activity 2

Fill in the blanks with the appropriate words.

1. If a patient doesn't understand what is happening, the medical professional needs to ________________ and make a ________________.
2. When medical professionals set up the ________________, they need to make sure they won't be interrupted, and there is plenty of privacy for the patient.
3. Warn patients before you give them bad news. Giving ________________ to the patient is extremely important.
4. Doctors and other medical professionals must show ________________ so that the patient feels understood and supported.
5. ________________ the patient's ________________ to make sure they know what their medical issue is and how serious it is.

Writing Activity

Imagine you are a patient about to receive bad news. Think about what things (words, actions, settings, etc.) would make the bad news easier to hear and accept. For example, talking to the doctor privately instead of in a place where other patients are listening might make you feel more comfortable. Write 4 or 5 sentences in the box provided.

When you're finished, share your writing with a partner or the class. Take notes of good points that other students make.

Listening Activity

Listen to a doctor deliver bad news to a patient. After you listen, answer the questions.

1. Why is Mr. Suda visiting his doctor now?

____

____

2. What is the first question the doctor asks Mr. Suda?

____

____

3. Why are the three health issues Mr. Suda was having?

____

____

4. What is the "good news" that the doctor mentions to Mr. Suda?

____

____

5. After delivering the bad news, as well as some potential good news, what does the doctor do?

____

____

Speaking Activity:The Bearer of Bad News

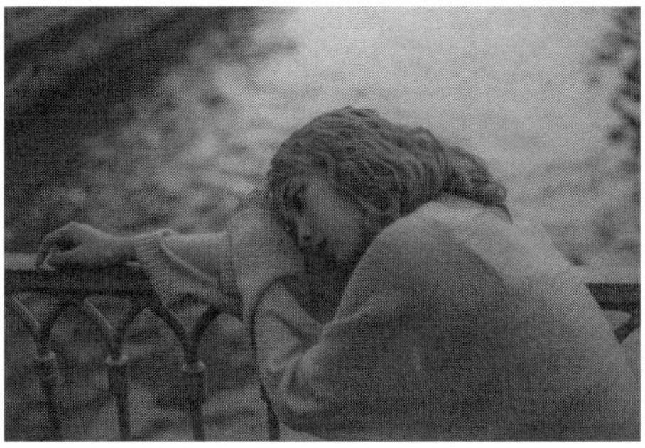

Practice these short "bad news" scripts with a partner. Take a deep breath and pause before you speak. After you deliver the bad news, think about how your partner may be feeling, and listen to their responses. When you finish, briefly talk about how you both felt giving and receiving bad news.

SCENE 1

Student 1: I'm sorry, but your car is being repossessed (撤去, てっきょ).
Student 2: But I don't have the money to make the payments!

SCENE 2

Student 1: I hate to tell you this, but there was a fire and your house burned down.
Student 2: What?! How could this happen?

SCENE 3

Student 1: Please have a seat. I'm sorry to say that the test results are positive.
Student 2: I don't understand. Diseases don't run in my family. This must be a mistake!

Now switch roles and repeat the exercise. Feel free to change the bad news and reactions, and add more dialogue to each scenario.

Discussion Questions

1. Share some bad news you recently heard or read about in the news or on the internet. What was the news? Who was involved? How did it make you feel when you heard the news? How did your family/friends react when they heard it?

2. Why do you think some people refuse to accept bad news? Think of a few reasons

and explain each one.

3. Giving bad news to patients is very difficult, and it is usually doctors who do it. Should doctors always be the person who gives patients bad news or should the responsibility be shared by others (nurses, specialists, etc.) ? Should the bad news always be verbal, or should letters be used in order to avoid conflict? What are the positive and negative points of verbal and written bad news?

Speaking Strategies: Presentation Slide Tips, Part 1

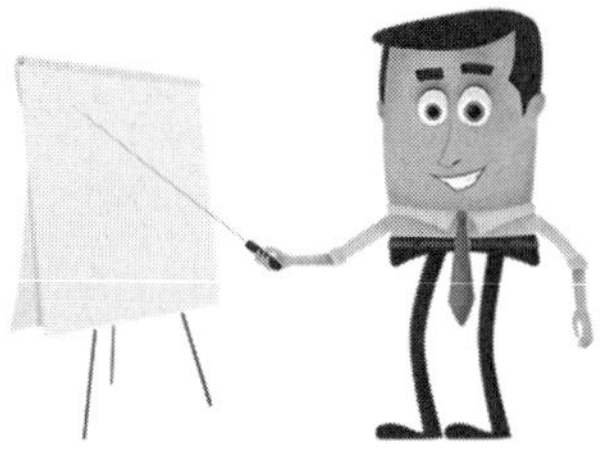

Long gone are the days of carrying around a bulky easel pad and a box full of different colored markers for presentations. Replacing the easel pad was the white board-on-wheels, but the box of markers was still needed. Then, in 1987, a breakthrough program was created that would change the face of presentations forever: Microsoft PowerPoint. Now available for both Windows and Mac, PowerPoint has become "the most widely used application for creating a computer-based presentation or slide show" (PowerPoint, n.d.) .

Since 1987, PowerPoint has gone through many changes, and other presentation programs were later introduced, such as Keynote and Prezi. Regardless of what program you use, these tips will help you make a clear, easy-to-follow presentation that will focus attention on you and your message.

Final Unit Assignment

Topic SPIKES Practice

Imagine you have to tell a patient she has breast cancer. Review SPIKES and explain each step. What would you do? Where would you hold the meeting? How long would the meeting be? What would you say? What would you not say? How would you react to different reactions from the patient (for example, crying, denial, anger, and silence) ? Be sure to go through each step of SPIKES and describe how you would approach each one.

UNIT 11

Caring for Children

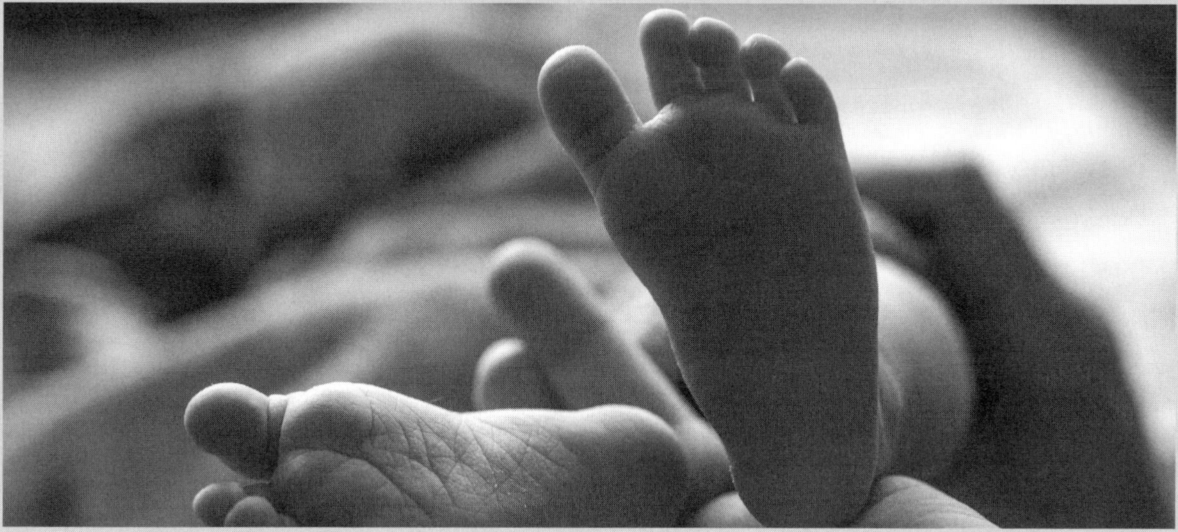

Medical Terms

1. pediatrics	小児科 (しょうにか)
2. mumps	おたふく風邪 (おたふくかぜ)
3. measles	麻疹 (はしか，ましん)
4. rubella	風疹 (ふうしん)
5. whooping cough	百日咳 (ひゃくにちぜき)
6. chicken pox	水疱瘡 (みずぼうそう)
7. tetanus	破傷風 (はしょうふう)
8. rash	発疹 (ほっしん)
9. malnutrition	栄養失調 (えいようしっちょう)
10. obesity	肥満 (ひまん)
11. diabetes	糖尿病 (とうにょうびょう)
12. hay fever	花粉症 (かふんしょう)
13. heat stroke	熱中症 (ねっちゅうしょう)
14. insomnia	不眠症 (ふみんしょう)
15. infancy	乳児期 (にゅうじき)
16. registration of birth	出生届 (しゅっせいとどけ)
17. toddler	よちよち歩き(あるき)の幼児(ようじ)
18. laparoscope	腹腔鏡 (ふくくうきょう)
19. endoscope	内視鏡 (ないしきょう)
20. gastroscope	胃 (い) カメラ

21. thermometer	体温計 (たいおんけい)
22. stethoscope	聴診器 (ちょうしんき)
23. self-adhesive bandage	絆創膏 (ばんそうこう)
24. gauze	ガーゼ
25. bandage	包帯 (ほうたい)
26. cast	ギプス
27. crutches	松葉杖 (まつばづえ)
28. rubber gloves	ゴム手袋 (てぶくろ)
29. syringe	注射器 (ちゅうしゃき)
30. operating table	手術台 (しゅじゅつだい)
31. scalpel	メス
32. splint	副木 (ふくぼく)
33. forceps	鉗子 (かんし)
34. tweezers	ピンセット
35. microscope	顕微鏡 (けんびきょう)
36. respirator	人工呼吸器 (じんこうこきゅうき)
37. unnatural death	変死 (へんし)
38. rigor mortis	死後硬直 (しごこうちょく)
39. epidemic	感染症 (かんせんしょう)
40. pandemic	パンデミック

Medical Terms: Practice

Match the medical terms (1-10) to their meanings (a-j).

1) ____ rash •	• a. infectious disease that causes fever and rash, mostly in children
2) ____ mumps •	• b. contagious viral disease that causes swelling of the cheeks
3) ____ pandemic •	• c. when an infectious disease spreads across the world
4) ____ forceps •	• d. red, itchy spots on a person's skin due to allergy or illness
5) ____ syringe •	• e. disease that affects the body' ability to produce insulin
6) ____ hay fever •	• f. tool used for injecting or withdrawing fluids with a hollow needle
7) ____ cast •	• g. protective shell of plaster used to protect broken bones
8) ____ chickenpox •	• h. the state of being extremely overweight
9) ____ obesity •	• i. allergy caused by dust or pollen
10) ____ diabetes •	• j. large tweezers or pincers used during surgery

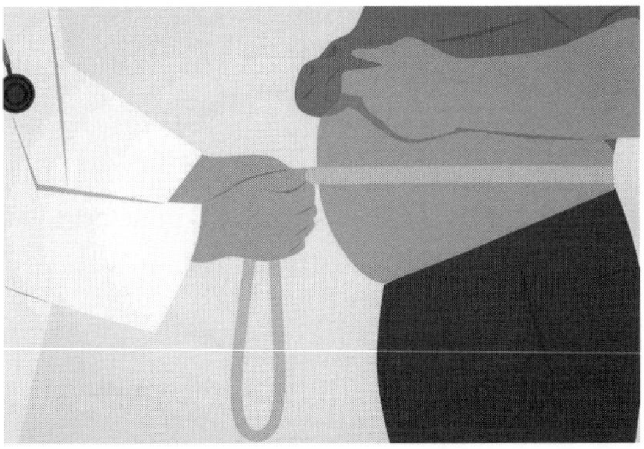

Obesity is the leading risk factor for type 2 diabetes.

0Grammar Review: The Imperative

The imperative tells people what to do. There are many ways to tell people what to do. You can give a person a strong command, you can give a person instructions for how to do something, you can give a person directions to a specific place, or you can give a person advice (which is basically a softer, gentler form of a command).

The imperative can be positive (affirmative) and negative. For a positive statement, the imperative is formed with the verb without a subject:

Look at children when you talk to them.
Write down all of the child's information.

For a negative statement, add "do not" or "don't" before the verb:

Don't interrupt child patients when they are talking.
Do not forget to smile when saying goodbye.

The imperative is often used on public signs, such as "Do not enter" (立入禁止, たちいりきんし), on forms, such as "Use a 2B pencil to mark the answer sheet," and on websites, like "Enter your password." The imperative is also used for instruction manuals and food products, like instant ramen noodles ("Add hot water and wait 3 minutes") .

Be careful when you use the imperative because it can sound harsh or rude:

Be quiet so I can check your pulse.
Put your toys away and listen to my instructions.
(*TIP: Add "please" to make these imperative statements a bit softer.*)

When used in the correct way, it can send positive and supportive messages:

Have a great day!
Call the clinic later so we can talk about your child's treatment.

Lastly, the imperative is a useful way to give someone advice:

Learn from the mistakes you make as a 1st-year medical student.
Be kind to all patients.

• Grammar Activity 1

Use the verbs in the box to make imperative statements.

forget	bring	rush	use	listen
answer	wrap	check	keep	be

1. Carefully ________________ to children when they're talking.

2. Don't ________________ a child's physical exam because they might get scared.

3. ________________ sensitive to the mothers' concerns.

4. ________________ the bandage on until the wound is completely healed.

5. Don't ________________ to talk to the child's father, as well. He may be nervous, too!

6. ________________ all of the parent's questions before they leave with their child.

7. ________________ to make sure the other children are being monitored in the waiting room.

8. ________________ the child's ankle tightly so he won't reinjure it.

9. ________________ new gloves for each patient.

10. ________________ all the forms that the child's parents or guardians need to read and sign.

• Grammar Activity 2

What advice would a medical professional give to children who are about to start junior high school? Write five sentences using the imperative.

1. ____

2. ____

3. ____

4. ____

5. ____

• Grammar Activity 3

Read your advice from **Activity 2** to a partner. After you finish, listen to your partner's advice, and write it down. Rank his or her advice from 1 to 5 (1 = not so good advice; 5 = great advice) .

Your partner's name: ____________________

His/Her advice:

Advice	Rank
1.	
2.	
3.	
4.	
5.	

Reading with Fushigi-chan: Child Development

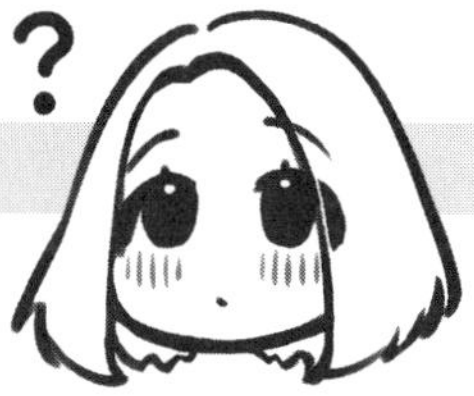

In Unit 8, you learned about pregnancy and some of the difficulties involved in giving birth, and may have had a chance to talk about some worries new parents might have. It is important for doctors, nurses, and other medical professionals to think about what is involved in having and raising a child because this information will help you provide better care to children and their parents. A lot of helpful information can be found in the studies of child development.

Crawling, taking a first step, learning to hold something, and saying a word for the first time are important parts of growing up. All of these parts can be put into categories called *developmental milestones*. While these milestones are worthy to become family members' social media highlights, they are very important to medical professionals because they tell them if a child is developing properly, or if there may be an issue with their development.

According to the Centers for Disease Control and Prevention (2022) , there are twelve milestones that should be monitored by parents and medical professionals. These twelve milestones start when a child is born and end at 5 years old, although

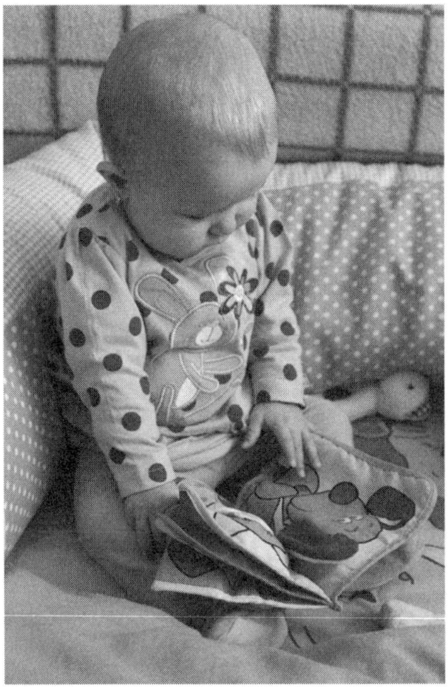

development doesn't stop there. Here are a few of the milestones with a summary of some important points to look for when examining a child patient:

- **2 months old**: At 2 months old, babies should be able to hold their heads up when lying on their stomach, look at people's faces, and smile when they are spoken to.
- **6 months old**: When babies are 6 months old, they should recognize familiar people, laugh, put things in their mouths, and support themselves with their hands when sitting.
- **12 months old**: At 12 months, children should understand the meaning of "no," pull themselves up to stand, and pick up small objects with their thumb and forefinger.
- **2 years old**: When children are around 2 years of age, they should be able to say two words together, use gestures, run, and eat with utensils.
- **4 years old**: A 4-year-old child should be able to play pretend, say basic sentences, hold a pencil between their fingers and thumb, and unbutton some of their shirt buttons.

It is very important not only for parents to be aware of developmental milestones, but also the doctors, nurses, and other medical professionals who are caring for them. If a child is not reaching one or more milestones or has somehow lost a previous skill that was once mastered, he or she needs to be evaluated by a doctor or multidisciplinary team of child specialists in order to give the child the help they need.

Children are amazing because they learn and grow so quickly and are able to adjust to a variety of situations. They are also extremely resilient and can overcome many challenges on their own or with gentle support from family, teachers, friends, and other people involved in their young lives. It is important for doctors, nurses, and other medical professionals to understand what a child should be able to do at their age and intervene if an issue arises.

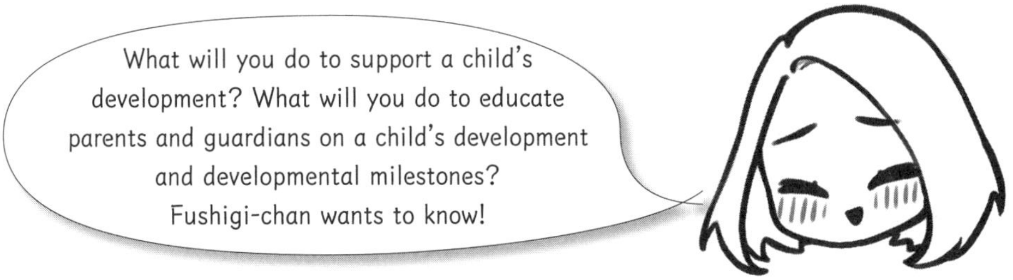

Reading Activity 1

Circle (T) if the statement is true or (F) if the statement is false.

1. A 12-month-old girl should be able to support herself with her hands. (T・F)
2. Only parents monitor their child's growth and development. (T・F)
3. There are twelve developmental milestones. (T・F)
4. 4-year-olds shouldn't be able to unbutton buttons. (T・F)
5. All children reach their developmental milestones. (T・F)

• Reading Activity 2

Fill in the blanks with the appropriate words.

1. If an issue arises with a child's development, medical professionals need to ______________ .
2. If a child has somehow ______________ a previous skill that was once mastered, he or she needs to be evaluated by a doctor or ______________ team.
3. Doctors and other medical professionals need to think about what is involved in ______________ and ______________ a child.

4. 12-month-old children should be able to pick up small objects with their __________ and __________ .

5. Medical professionals needs to educate __________ and __________ on a child's development and developmental milestones.

Writing Activity

Children are often afraid to go to a hospital or clinic. What ways could children feel more comfortable? Think of ways to create a comfortable, fun, and supportive atmosphere for children, and write your ideas below. When you're finished, create a poster or brochure advertising a new children's clinic that reflects your ideas. Feel free to use color markers, pictures, stickers, shapes—anything to make it fun for children.

When you're finished, share your writing, poster or brochure with a partner or the class.

Listening Activity

Listen to a nurse talk to a child patient. While you're listening, fill in the blanks below.

1. My name is Erika, and I'm a ______________ nurse. " ______________ " is just a big word that means I help children.

2. If it's ok with you, I'd like to do a couple of tests to make sure your body is ______________ and ______________ .

3. First I'm going to put this on your chest. It's called a ______________ , and it helps me to listen to the ______________ of your body.

4. I can see you're ______________ a bit, so I'm going to ask your mom to hold your hand while I do this, OK Saori?

5. There, all done! You did a great job. Next, I need to check your ______________ , so I'm going to have you lie down on your back for me. Mom, can you lay Saori down on the table while I prepare the next ______________ ?

Speaking Activity: Giving Directions

In the **Grammar** section, you learned about the imperative form of verbs, and how you can use the imperative to give directions or instructions to patients. For this next exercise, you are going to work with a partner.

Student 1 is the clinic doctor, nurse, or receptionist. Use the map at the end of the unit, choose a location, and then give your partner directions to the clinic. Make sure you use the imperative (for example, "Turn left," "Cross the street," or "Go straight") .

Student 2 is a new patient calling for directions. Use the map on the next page to locate the clinic while listening to the directions. Confirm the directions before ending the call. When the conversation has ended, check to see if the correct location was found.

Use this mini script to start the phone conversation:

Student 1: Good morning. Health Clinic.

Student 2: Good morning. My name is ______________ and I have an appointment with Dr. Hayashi at 10:30.

Student 1: Oh, good morning, Mr./Ms. ______________ . This is ______________ .

How can I help you?

Student 2: I'm looking forward to my first appointment at your clinic, but I'm afraid I don't know how to get there.

Student 1: I see. Will you arrive at the bus terminal or the train station?

Student 2: I'll be arriving at the train station.

Student 1: OK, in that case, you first want to take the North exit. Next, ... (*give directions to your clinic*) .

Student 2 Map

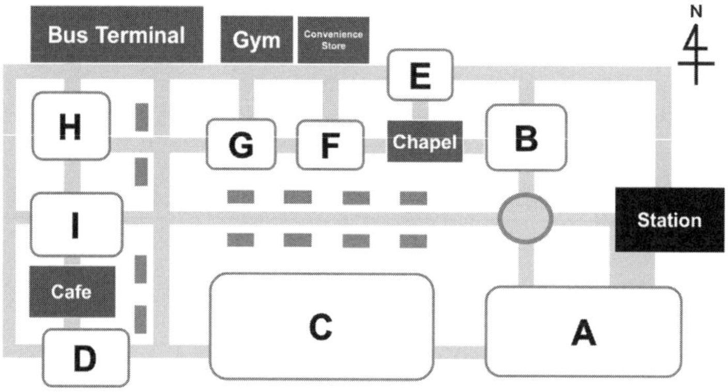

Clinic location: ______

When you finish, switch roles. Student 2 will choose a *new* location for the clinic and give directions to Student 1. You can also add other locations, such as a pharmacy or medical school.

Discussion Questions

1. What are the main differences between adult patients and child patients? List ten differences with your partner or small group.

2. When you become a doctor, nurse, or other medical professional, would you prefer working with children or adults? Why?

3. What do you think are some good points about working in a children's clinic or children's ward? What do you think are some of the challenges?

Speaking Strategies: Presentation Structure, Part I

Some would agree that the beginning of anything—a song, a book, a new job, a friendship, a conversation, a meal, a lesson—is the most important part, as it sets up what is to come. The same can be said for a presentation, a classroom discussion, or a formal debate. How you begin will prepare your audience for what they are about to see and hear. A sound structure to your presentation, discussion or debate will help you create a persuasive and memorable message for your audience.

Final Unit Assignment

Topic Caring for pediatric patients

According to the World Health Organization (WHO) , global obesity rates have tripled since 1975. Unsurprisingly, child obesity is also on the rise in almost every country around the world. Although countries like Japan have a lower percentage of obese children (4.99% boys, 1.73% girls) compared to countries like America (23.29% boys, 19.47% girls) , the numbers are still concerning (World Obesity, 2022) .

You are a group of medical professionals who have been brought together to present their suggestions to the Board of Education, as well as to government officials, parent groups, and student representatives. Present, discuss, debate, or write about the following topic:

All schools at every level (from day care to graduate school) should (or should not) make it mandatory for students to exercise 30 minutes a day and have their weight monitored every month.

Come up with three reasons why this is a good idea, or three reasons it's not a good idea. If this is a class debate, one group will come up with points that support this idea, and the other team will come up with negative points. If you can access the internet, find research, political opinions, possible dangers, etc., and use them to support your position. At the end of the presentations or debates, the instructor or a student judge will decide which argument was more persuasive.

Speaking Activity: Giving Directions

Student 1 Map

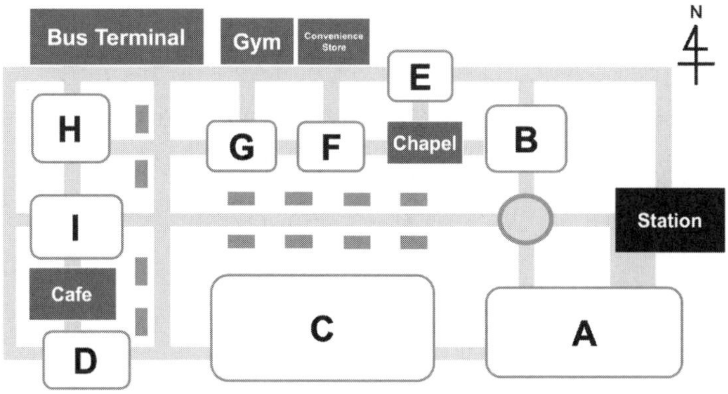

UNIT

12 Caring for Adults

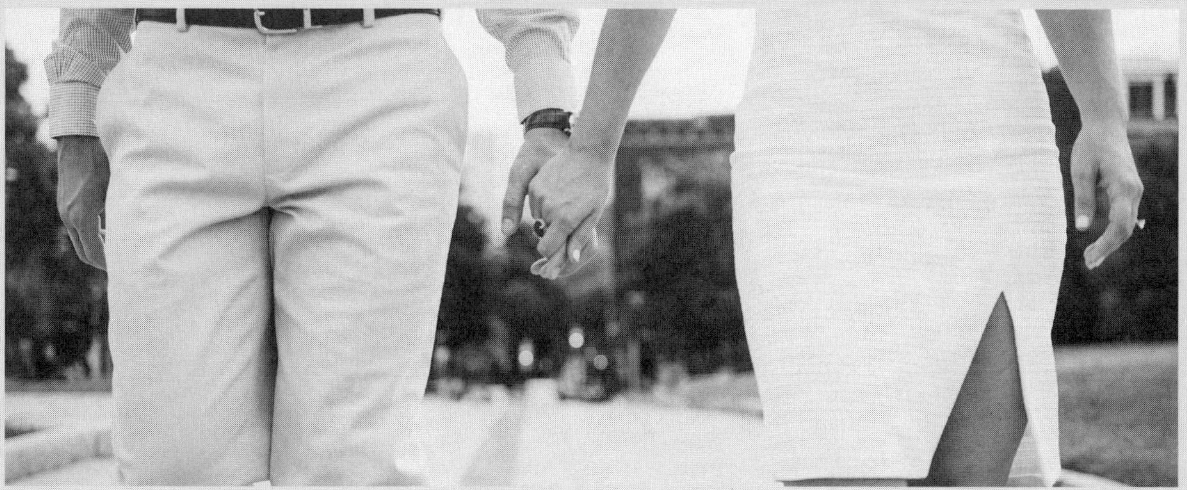

Medical Terms

1. intravenous drip (IV)	点滴 (てんてき)
2. cosmetic surgery	美容整形 (びようせいけい)
3. incision	切開 [術] (せっかい [じゅつ])
4. hypodermic injection	皮下注射 (ひかちゅうしゃ)
5. laser procedure	レーザー治療 (ちりょう)
6. physical therapy	理学療法 (りがくりょうほう)
7. occupational therapy	作業療法 (さぎょうりょうほう)
8. surgery	手術 (しゅじゅつ)
9. anesthesia	麻酔 (ますい)
10. alternative medicine	代替医療 (だいたいいりょう)
11. holistic medicine	全人的医学 (ぜんじんてきいがく)
12. hysterectomy	子宮摘出術 (しきゅうてきしゅつじゅつ)
13. vasectomy	精管切除 (せいかんせつじょ), パイプカット
14. tubal litigation	卵管結紮 (らんかんけっさつ)
15. cesarean section	帝王切開 (ていおうせっかい)
16. chemotherapy	化学療法 (かがくりょうほう)
17. blood transfusion	輸血 (ゆけつ)
18. coronary bypass	冠動脈 (かんどうみゃく) バイパス
19. artificial respiration	人工呼吸 (じんこうこきゅう)
20. gastrectomy	胃切除術 (いせつじょじゅつ)
21. immunotherapy	免疫療法 (めんえきりょうほう)

22. intravenous injection	静脈 [内] 注射 (じょうみゃく [ない] ちゅうしゃ)
23. gene therapy	遺伝子療法 (いでんしりょうほう)
24. intubation	挿管 (そうかん)
25. traction	牽引 (けんいん)
26. organ transplant	臓器移植 (ぞうきいしょく)
27. ostectomy	骨切除[術] (こつせつじょ[じゅつ])
28. radio therapy	放射線療法 (ほうしゃせんりょうほう)
29. intramuscular injection	筋肉注射 (きんにくちゅうしゃ)
30. serotherapy	血清療法 (けっせいりょうほう)
31. thermotherapy	温熱療法 (おんねつりょうほう)
32. sterilization	避妊手術 (ひにんしゅじゅつ), 消毒 (しょうどく), 殺菌 (さっきん)
33. nutrition therapy	栄養療法 (えいようりょうほう)
34. urethral catheterization	尿道 (にょうどう) カテーテル法 (ほう)
35. dialysis	透析 (とうせき)
36. disinfection	消毒 (しょうどく)
37. first aid	応急処置 (おうきゅうしょち)
38. staples	ステープル
39. suture	縫合 (ほうごう)
40. resuscitate	蘇生 (そせい) させる

Medical Terms: Practice

Use the medical terms to complete the sentences.

1) A small ______________ needs to be made near the patient's navel in order to repair the hernia.

2) ______________ is a form of male birth control that involves cutting and sealing the tubes that carry sperm.

3) If your appendix bursts (ruptures) , you will need ______________ to remove it as soon as possible.

4) The doctor suggested ______________ to the cancer patient, but surprisingly she declined the treatment.

5) Every person should know how to deliver basic ______________ . You never know when an accident could happen, so you should always be prepared to help!

6) After my sports injury, I had to undergo ______________ to relieve my pain and help improve my movements.

7) After seeing all the beautiful men and women on television, I understand why many people want ______________ ______________ to change their appearance.

8) When my sister fell off her bicycle, the doctor had to ______________ the large cut in her leg.

9) An ______________ ______________ delivers important vitamins and nutrients to directly into patients' bloodstreams.

10) Before an operation, it is important to ask patients if they have ever had an allergic reaction to ______________ .

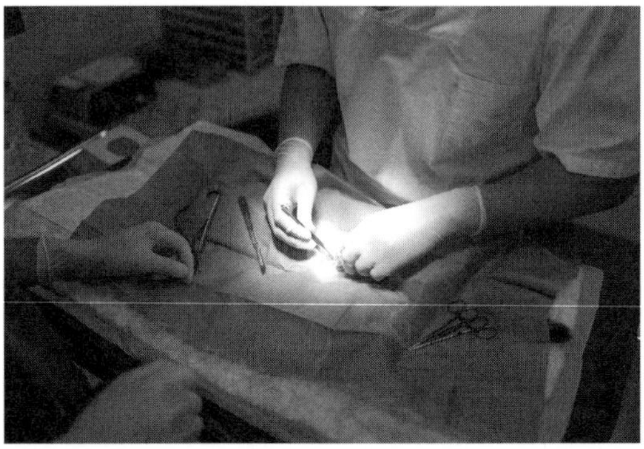

Grammar Review: Modals

In **Unit 10**, you learned about the auxiliary verb "had." *Auxiliary* verb is a grammar phrase that means "helping verb," meaning it helps the main verb send a clear message to the reader or listener. There are several types of modals that we'll look at in this unit. Here is a list of the most common modals, their meanings, and some example sentences.

modal verb (positive and negative)	meaning	example sentence
Can / Can't	1) Ability/inability 2) informal request 3) possibility or impossibility (*can't*)	1) I can perform a blood test. 2) Can you check on that patient? 3) The lump in his arm can be benign or cancerous.
Could	1) Asking for permission 2) polite request 3) suggestion 4) possibility	1) Could I have a new lab coat? 2) Could you pass me some bandages? 3) You could try to reschedule surgery for Monday. 4) It could be food poisoning.
Must / Mustn't	1) obligation 2) deduce (draw a conclusion) 3) prohibition (*mustn't*)	1) You must contact me immediately if the pain returns. 2) Your nausea must have been caused by the new medication. 3) You mustn't perform surgery if you haven't slept.
Have to / Don't have to	1) obligation 2) not necessary to do (*don't have to*)	1) You have to wear gloves during surgery. 2) You don't have to wear a lab coat during Medical English classes.
May	1) polite request 2) possibility	1) May I have the patient's chart, please? 2) Dr. Sato may have left her glasses in the cafeteria.
Might	1) possibility 2) suggestion	1) The patient might be 10 minutes late for his appointment. 2) You might want to research this area before going to the medical conference.
Should / Ought to	1) advice 2) regret (*should + have + verb*)	1) You should exercise regularly. 2) I should have rescheduled this surgery.

• Grammar Activity 1

Complete the dialogue with the correct modal verb.

Dr. Smith: As you can see from your recent test results, your cholesterol is very high. ____________ I ask about any recent lifestyle changes?

Ms. Nakamura: Well, since my last physical exam, you said I ____________ exercise more regularly, but the opposite has happened.

Dr. Smith: Are you stressed at work?

Ms. Nakamura: Yes! I ____________ ____________ reduced my work hours, but actually I work overtime almost every day.

Dr. Smith: ____________ you exercise on the weekends?

Ms. Nakamura: I tried, but it's difficult because the kids always want to eat fast food and relax with me. I ____________ ____________ be stricter, but honestly fast food and relaxing with my kids is the only break I get from work.

Dr. Smith: I understand. There's nothing wrong with rewarding ourselves once in a while, but you ____________ want to talk to them about the entire family eating healthier.

Ms. Nakamura: You're right. I ____________ ____________ done that sooner. Do I ____________ ____________ take medication to reduce my cholesterol?

Dr. Smith: I ____________ prescribe you a low dosage statin, which will help reduce your cholesterol, but you ____________ consider changing some of the unhealthy lifestyle choices.

Ms. Nakamura: I ____________ consider starting medication, but first let me see if I can make some drastic lifestyle changes. Thank you, doctor.

• Grammar Activity 2

Rewrite these statements using modals to make them sound more polite.

1. Hand me the scalpel.

   ____

2. Review this paper for me.

   ____

3. Meet me in the library.

____

4. Study for the next medical English test.

____

5. Learn from your mistakes.

____

• Grammar Activity 3

Read the problems, and then offer some advice.

1. Problem: The medical student is always late for 1st period English class.

   Advice: ____

2. Problem: The nurse is having trouble reading his patients' charts.

   Advice: ____

3. Problem: I don't know which hospital I should choose to have my exam.

   Advice: ____

4. Problem: She's afraid to have surgery.

   Advice: ____

5. Problem: My husband is gaining weight, but he hates eating vegetables.

   Advice: ____

Reading with Fushigi-chan: Adult Health Issues

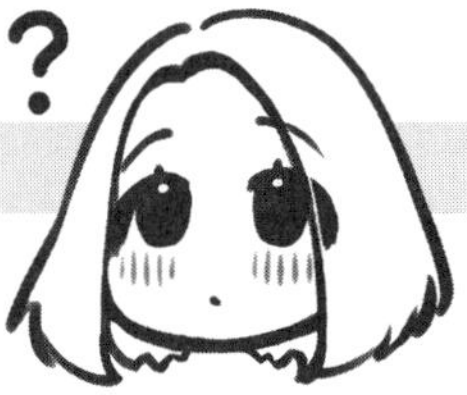

Readers of this textbook are probably medical students or working professionals, and therefore most likely in one of the various stages of adulthood. Most children hardly ever think about health issues unless they are born with or develop one during childhood, and usually have a false sense of invincibility. Adults, however, realize that they are not invincible, and begin to think about medical issues as they grow older.

Before looking into some of the medical concerns, it's important to look at some of the health issues many adults face. When one becomes an adult, they usually begin to work a full-time job. Many jobs are sedentary—in other words, the job is done sitting down for long periods of time. Sedentary lifestyles are inactive lifestyles, which lead to weight issues (overweight and obesity) , as well as nutrition issues (eating more fast food or skipping meals) . Mental health is also a concern for many adults, especially if their job or relationship is a source of severe stress. Habits, such as drinking alcohol excessively, smoking, and doing drugs, all have a tremendous impact on health. Lastly, the environment—the place adults live and work—can affect mental and physical health (for example, pollution, violence, and difficulty accessing health services) .

One of the main health issues for adults is heart disease. While some heart problems are hereditary, or passed from parents to children, others can be prevented with certain lifestyle changes and medication. There are two interesting risk factors connected to heart disease: age is a factor (more adults suffer from heart disease than children) , as well as gender (men are more likely to have heart issues than women) .

Cancer, of course, begins to enter people's minds when they become adults. Cancer is the new, abnormal, and uncontrollable division of cells in the body leading to growths known as tumors. Although children can get cancer, chances increase when a person becomes an adult. According to the National Cancer Institute (2022) , common cancers include lung, bladder, and thyroid cancer, and some are found in men (prostate cancer) while others affect mostly women (breast cancer) . As mentioned in a previous unit, early detection is key to helping patients overcome their cancer diagnosis.

Caring for adult patients is much different than caring for children or elderly patients, and, in many ways, it is a much more complex process. The best way doctors, nurses, and other medical professionals can support adult patients is to listen to them, try to understand their life situation (family, work, lifestyle habits, and stresses) , and use medical knowledge to offer the best guidance and treatment.

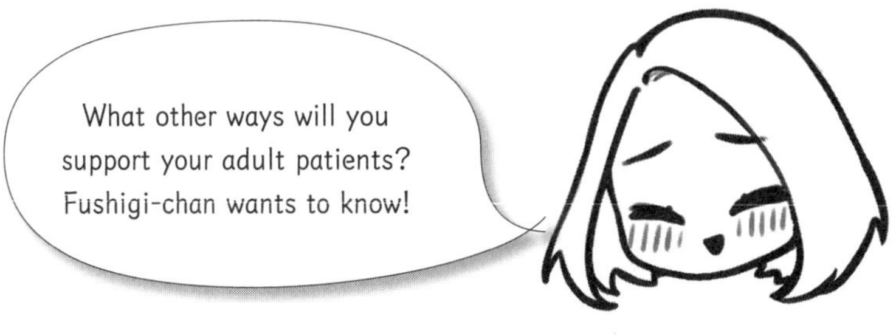

• Reading Activity 1

Circle (T) if the statement is true or (F) if the statement is false.

1. The best way a doctor can help adult patients is to give them medicine. (T・F)
2. Age and gender are risk factors for adult patients. (T・F)
3. Habits like drinking alcohol only slightly impact a person's health. (T・F)
4. Children don't have to worry about health issues until they're older. (T・F)
5. Lifestyle changes can help some heart problems that are hereditary. (T・F)

• Reading Activity 2

Fill in the blanks with the appropriate words.

1. Most children usually never think about serious health issues because they have a feeling ______________ . Like a superhero, they believe nothing can hurt them.
2. A bad environment can impact a patient's mental and physical health, such as ______________ , ______________ , and ______________ ______________ ______________ ______________ .
3. Some heart problems can be improved or prevented with ______________ ______________ and ______________ .
4. A job that is done sitting down for long periods of time with very little movement is called ______________ work.
5. One of the best ways a medical professional can support a patient is to understand their life— ______________ , ______________ , ______________ ______________ , and ______________ —and use their medical knowledge to offer the best guidance and advice.

Writing Activity

The diagram below is called a Venn Diagram. You can use a Venn Diagram to look at two topics and see their differences, but also what similarities they share. Think about adult patients and child patients. What different needs do they have? What similar needs do they have? How will treatment differ? Work alone or with a partner and write some similarities and differences in the diagram.

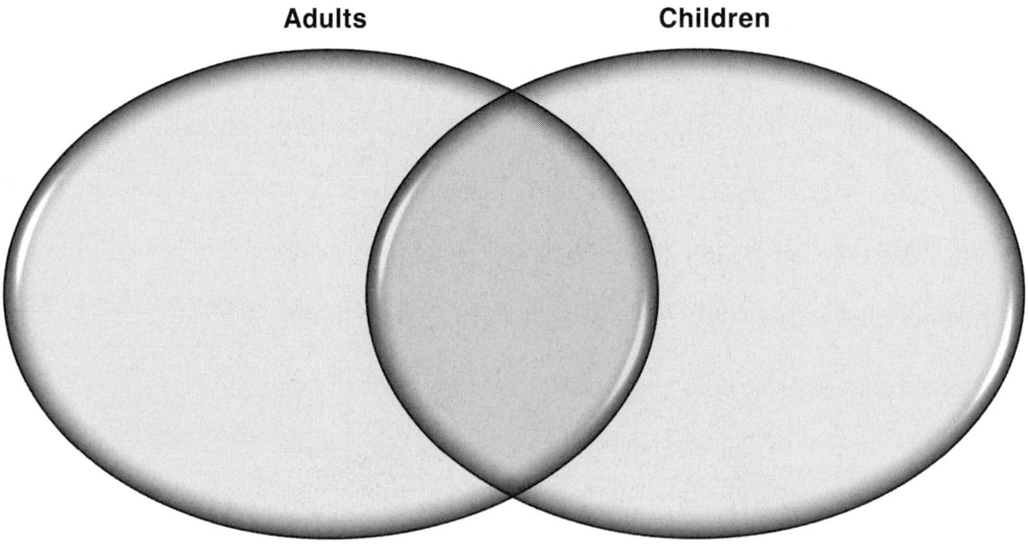

When you're finished, share your ideas with a new partner and see what ideas you can add to your diagram.

Listening Activity

Listen to an adult discuss an experience with a doctor and nurses. After you finish listening to the speaker, answer the questions below.

Question 1: When the speaker was a child, how did she communicate with the medical staff?

Question 2: Were her experiences as a child positive or negative?

Question 3: Why did she take her 2-year-old son to the Emergency Room?

Question 4: What was the main concern of the doctor and nurses?

Question 5: What does the speaker hope doctors and nurses do when treating all patients?

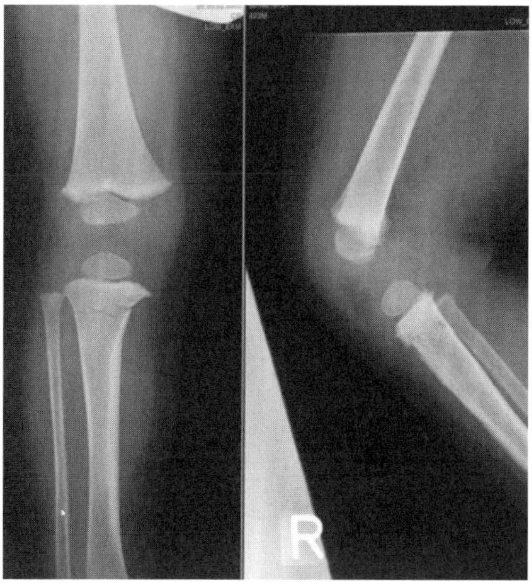

Speaking Activity

Unlike children, adults are independent and capable of making decisions on their own. Unfortunately, not all these decisions are what's best for their mental and physical health.

Look at the two cards below. Each set of cards contain roles for a medical professional (doctor, nurse, etc.) and patient. Work with a partner and decide who will play each role. After you choose, role play each situation in this way:

- First, the medical professional presents the test results (written in quotation marks: " ") and offers advice (written in *italics*) ;
- The patient then gives an excuse as to why they cannot follow the medical professional's advice. This can be done casually, reluctantly, or aggressively.
- The medical professional should then respond with more advice and/or a warning.
- Finally, the patient can either accept the advice or make one more excuse. At this point, switch roles and do Scene 2. The roles can also stay the same for Scene 2, and then you can switch roles and do both scenes again.

Scene 1: Medical Professional

"Regarding your recent panic attacks, your tests results have come back negative, but this is a possible sign of heart disease. (*Offer advice on doing exercise, limiting smoking/drinking, and eating healthy foods*) . It could also be a sign of anxiety. (*Suggest seeing a mental health therapist*) .

Scene 1: Patient

Give an excuse against exercise, etc. (Example: "But I don't smoke that much!")

or

Give an excuse against seeing a mental health therapist. (Example: "But I'm not crazy! Only crazy people see therapists.")

Scene 2: Medical Professional

"I have your physical exam results. Your complaints about recent bloating could be because of your diet. Are you eating too much food during each meal or perhaps drinking too much water? (*Give advice about a balanced diet or keeping a food journal*) . This could also be a more serious sign of cancer—colon, ovarian, stomach or even pancreatic cancer." (*Recommend multiple cancer screening tests*) .

Scene 2: Patient

Disagree with the medical professional's suggestion about food and drinks. (Example: "There's no problem with my diet! I eat things like _____.")

or

Refuse cancer screening. (Example: "I don't have time to go through all those tests. Besides, if I have cancer, I don't want to know about it! We all have to die sometime.")

Discussion Questions

1. According to the National Center for Chronic Disease Prevention and Health Promotion (2022) , in the Unites States 96 million adults have prediabetes, almost 31 million adults smoke cigarettes, and 74% of adults are overweight or obese. Discuss three strategies you will use to improve the health of your adult clients.

2. Some countries have social problems related to overwork. Overworking can lead to

higher stress levels, unhealthy habits, such as excessive alcohol consumption and smoking, and, in some extreme cases, depression, anxiety, and suicide. What do you think of this issue, and what can doctors, nurses, and other medical professionals do to support patients experiencing overwork?

3. In the last chapter, you learned about child patients. When children are stressed (from school, relationships, etc.) , the parents usually become stressed. There are some ways that parents and children can reduce stress together, such as playing games, dancing, and even snuggling. If you're a medical professional and an adult patient asks you about family stress, what are three suggestions you would give him or her?

Speaking Strategies: Presentation Structure, Part II

In the previous unit, the introduction of a presentation or speech was covered. In this unit, we will continue with a sound structure of a presentation (speech or academic written assignment). From the introduction, you can naturally transition into the main part of your presentation, which consists of your main points. In academic writing, this main section is often referred to as the "body" of the essay. These main points contain two parts: explaining the main point and providing support.

Final Unit Assignment

Topic Alternative Medicine

Alternative medicine and treatments have become more popular. Users of Chinese medicine, acupuncture, homeopathy, and body movement therapies have increased, and while this is not a bad thing, what is troubling is that many people use alternative medicine and treatment instead of going to the hospital and taking prescribed medicine. According to Nahin, et al. (2010) ,

> 19.3% of adults (38.3 million) did not use conventional care in a 12 month period, although 39.5% of these individuals (14.7 million) reported having one or more problems with their health. Of those not using conventional care, 24.8% (9.5 million) used alternative medicine.

Research an alternative medicine and present your findings in an essay or presentation. What is the medicine or treatment, and why are people attracted to it? What ways can medical professionals also promote conventional care options?

UNIT

13 Caring for the Elderly

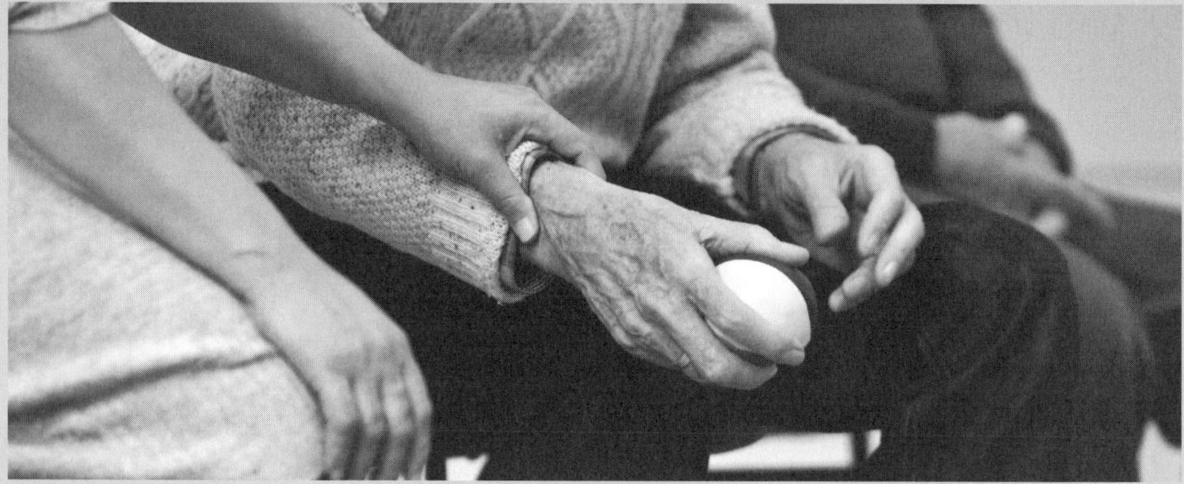

Medical Terms

1. health management	健康管理 (けんこうかんり)
2. physical exam	健康診断 (けんこうしんだん)
3. geriatrics	老年医学 (ろうねんいがく)
4. elderly	高齢者 (こうれいしゃ)
5. birth rate	出生率 (しゅっせいりつ)
6. aging society	高齢化社会 (こうれいかしゃかい)
7. average life expectancy	平均余命 (へいきんよめい)
8. carcinogen	発がん物質 (はつがんぶっしつ)
9. disabled / handicapped person	障害者 (しょうがいしゃ)
10. caretaker	家庭訪問員 (かていほうもんいん)
11. social worker	ソーシャルワーカー
12. at-home care	在宅看護 (ざいたくかんご)
13. nursing home	介護施設 (かいごしせつ)
14. hospice	ホスピス
15. national health insurance	健康保険 (けんこうほけん)
16. private hospital	私立病院 (しりつびょういん)
17. public hospital	公立病院 (こうりつびょういん)
18. quarantine	検疫 (けんえき)
19. vaccination	予防接種 (よぼうせっしゅ)
20. eating habits	食習慣 (しょくしゅうかん)

21. vegetarian	菜食主義者(さいしょくしゅぎしゃ)
22. heavy smoker	愛煙家 (あいえんか)
23. drug addict	麻薬中毒者(まやくちゅうどくしゃ)
24. alcoholic	アルコール中毒患者(ちゅうどくかんじゃ)
25. Alzheimer's disease	アルツハイマー病 (びょう)
26. dementia	認知症 (にんちしょう)
27. Parkinson's disease	パーキンソン病 (びょう)
28. childhood	幼児期 (ようじき), 児童期 (じどうき)
29. puberty	思春期 (ししゅんき)
30. adolescence	青年期 (せいねんき)
31. child-bearing age	出産適齢期(しゅっさんてきれいき)
32. rebellious stage	反抗期 (はんこうき)
33. adulthood	成人期 (せいじんき)
34. beginning of menstrual cycle	初経 (しょけい), 初潮 (しょちょう)
35. maternity leave	産休 (さんきゅう)
36. menopause	更年期 (こうねんき)
37. old age	老年期 (ろうねんき)
38. registration of death	死亡届 (しぼうとどけ)
39. medical malpractice	医療過誤 (いりょうかご)
40. organ donor	臓器提供者(ぞうきていきょうしゃ)

Medical Terms: Practice

Match the medical terms（1-10）to their Japanese translations（a-j）.

1) menopause •	• a. 健康管理（けんこうかんり）
2) puberty •	• b. 健康診断（けんこうしんだん）
3) heavy smoker •	• c. 愛煙家（あいえんか）
4) health management •	• d. 思春期（ししゅんき）
5) carcinogen •	• e. 発がん物質（はつがんぶっしつ）
6) physical exam •	• f. 高齢化社会（こうれいかしゃかい）
7) quarantine •	• g. 医療過誤（いりょうかご）
8) disabled person •	• h. 検疫（けんえき）
9) aging society •	• i. 障害者（しょうがいしゃ）
10) medical malpractice •	• j. 更年期（こうねんき）

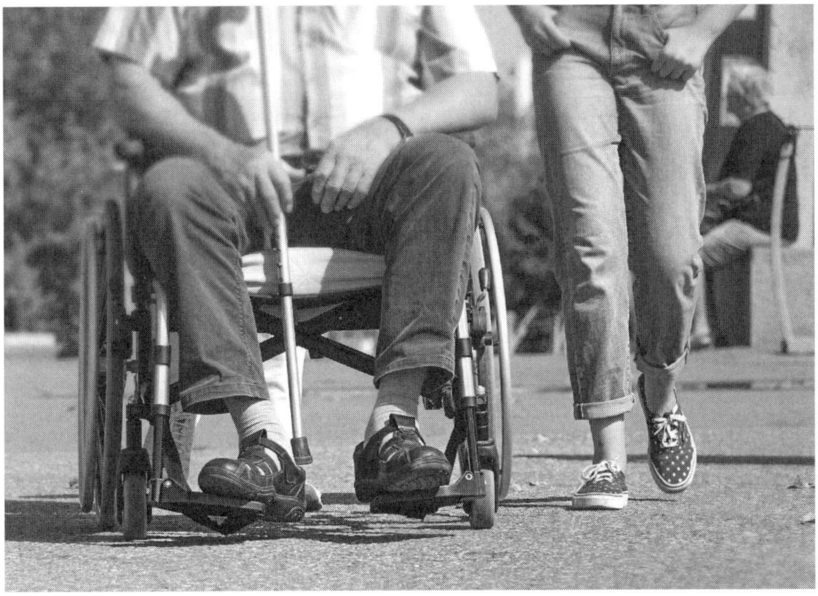

Grammar Review: Present Progressive

The present progressive is also known as the present continuous, which might help understand how to use it. We use the present progressive to show an action or event that is in progress. In other words, the action or event started but has not finished yet or is continuing at the same time the speaker is speaking.

Making the present progressive is easy—use the present form of the verb *be* plus a present participle (the -ing form of a verb, or -ing participle) .

I **am** study*ing* English right now.
We **are** read*ing* the new medical English textbook.

Remember that contractions are usually used when having a conversation and in informal writing.

I'**m** study*ing* English right now.
We'**re** read*ing* the new medical English textbook.

Although the present progressive is used when the action is ongoing in the present, this form can also be used to talk about a planned activity or event in the future.

I **am** mov*ing* to America next year for a medical internship.
The bullet train to Tokyo **is** depart*ing* in 10 minutes.

To make the negative form of the present progressive, add *not* after the present form of the verb *be*.

They **are not** listen*ing* to the teacher.
Sara'**s not** (or Sara **isn't**) eat*ing* lunch with us today.

Lastly, we can also use the present progressive to ask questions:

Are you look*ing* for the new lecture room?
Is Sara eat*ing* lunch with us today?

• Grammar Activity 1

Use the words to make sentences and questions in the present progressive.

1. The professor / lecture about elderly care.

2. Your partner / explain the lab procedures in English?

3. Two students / give a presentation about drawing blood.

4. You / attend the seminar on heart disease?

5. I / move to Germany for a 3-month internship.

• Grammar Activity 2

Read the blog and complete the sentences by circling the correct choices. The present progressive and other tenses are used.

My Medical School Blog

It's Thursday morning, and I am so (**sleepy/sleeping**). I (**am sitting/sit**) in class (**listen/listening**) to a lecture on caring for the elderly, but my eyes won't stay open! In order to stay awake, I (**write/am writing**) this blog now. I (**hoping/hope**) it's interesting!

The student next to me (**is watching/watches**) a video on his phone and (**taps/is tapping**) his finger on the desk, and it is (**annoying/annoyed**). The professor (**writes/is writing**) on the whiteboard, but his letters are too small. I can't (**reading/read**) anything on the board! On top of this, the air conditioner (**is running/runs**) at the highest level, but it (**is freezing/had been freezing**) in here.

Some students (**are sleeping/is sleeping**) , but most of them (**are taking/takes**) notes. I (**am going/go**) to Universal Studios Japan tomorrow with my friends, so I need to start (**focus/focusing**) on today's lesson.

Thank you for (**read/reading**) my blog. (**Wish/Wishing**) me luck!

• Grammar Activity 3

Look at the picture of some 1st-year medical students working on a project in class. Describe what they're doing using the present progressive.

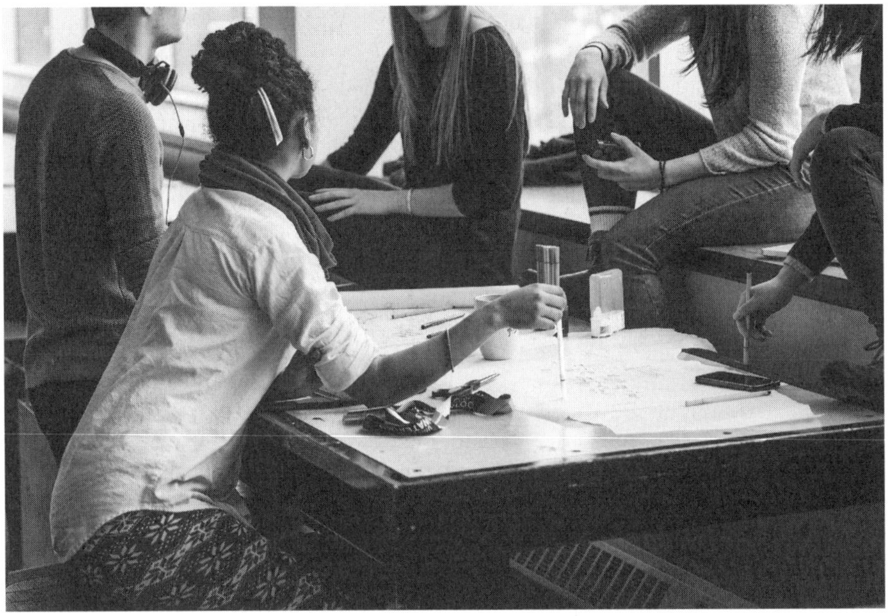

1. The guy in the gray shirt __________ __________________ headphones.

2. The two girls on the right __________ __________________ on the window sill.

3. The girl in the front __________ __________________ a scarf.

4. The girl in the middle of the picture __________ __________________ to the girl with the scarf.

5. The girl on the right __________ __________________ a pen.

Reading with Fushigi-chan: Elderly Health Issues

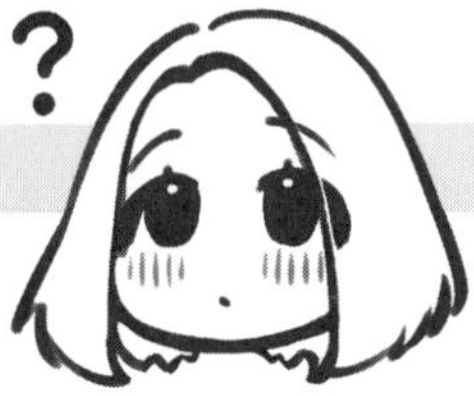

Most countries will probably have an expression like "Respect your elders." In some cultures, older members of the group are revered and celebrated. Elderly people, also known as the aged, senior citizens or simply "old people," are a special group with very special medical needs.

According to the World Health Organization (2022), "Most developed world countries

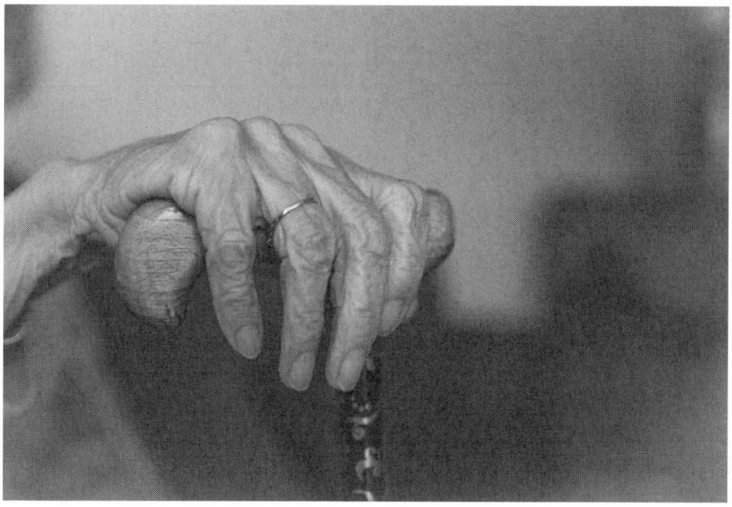

have accepted the chronological age of 65 years as a definition of 'elderly' or older person." The branch of medicine that deals with the care of the elderly, as well as prevention and treatment of diseases related to the elderly, is called geriatrics, and a specialist in geriatrics is called a geriatrician.

Because of their advanced age, there are many ailments and diseases that affect the elderly population. The most prevalent are chronic health issues—issues that last for a long time or are constantly a problem. Examples of chronic health conditions are diabetes, heart disease, and cancer. Cognitive health, including mental health, are also concerns. The most common is Alzheimer's Disease, a form of dementia. Physical issues are also a problem, especially accidental falls, which many elderly people experience. Other issues include vision and hearing loss, tooth decay and loss, and urinary incontinence (loss of bladder control) .

Labella, et al. (2011) explain there are "challenges in caring for this patient population [that] include dosing medications safely, preventing delirium and accidental falls, and providing adequate pain control." There are other factors that can also make caring for the elderly challenging, and these may come as a surprise to many doctors, nurses, and other medical professionals. As mentioned above, hearing loss and a loss of intellectual abilities can make things like gaining patient consent or ensuring a patient remembers to take prescribed medication an enormous struggle. In addition, the stress can become too much for some caregivers, who are usually family members who must take care of elderly relatives at home, and sometimes this frustration shows during medical visits.

Many countries are struggling with an aging population, and the World Health

Organization (2017) estimates that 22% of the world's population will be over 60 by 2050. There has never been a more urgent time to provide appropriate medical care and support to this important group of people. Remembering to speak slowly and clearly to elderly patients, checking often for understanding, and being compassionate and empathetic are keys to establishing a good relationship with your elderly patients and helping them with their unique medical needs.

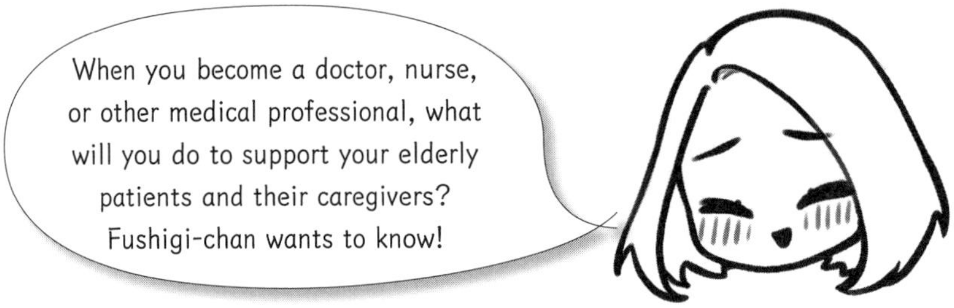

• Reading Activity 1

Answer these questions about elderly care.

1. What are some of the issues facing elderly people?

____

____

2. What are some of the challenges medical professionals face when providing care for the elderly?

____

____

3. How can medical professionals make elderly patients feel more comfortable and more willing to participate in treatment programs?

____

____

4. What problems do some caregivers have when caring for elderly family members?

____

____

5. Why are accidental falls so prevalent (common) among the elderly?

____

____

• Reading Activity 2

Fill in the blanks with the missing words.

1. By the year 2050, __________________ of the world's population may be over __________________ .

2. The branch of medicine that deals with the prevention and treatment of diseases related to the elderly is called __________________ , and a specialist in this field is called a __________________ .

3. Medical professionals must remember to speak __________________ and __________________ to elderly patients.

4. Challenges in caring for elderly patients include __________________ __________________ safely, preventing __________________ , and providing adequate __________________ control.

5. __________________ and __________________ are keys to establishing a good relationship with elderly patients.

Writing Activity

What are some issues with an aging population? Using the information in the reading section, as well as your own knowledge and ideas, write 4 or 5 issues in the box provided.

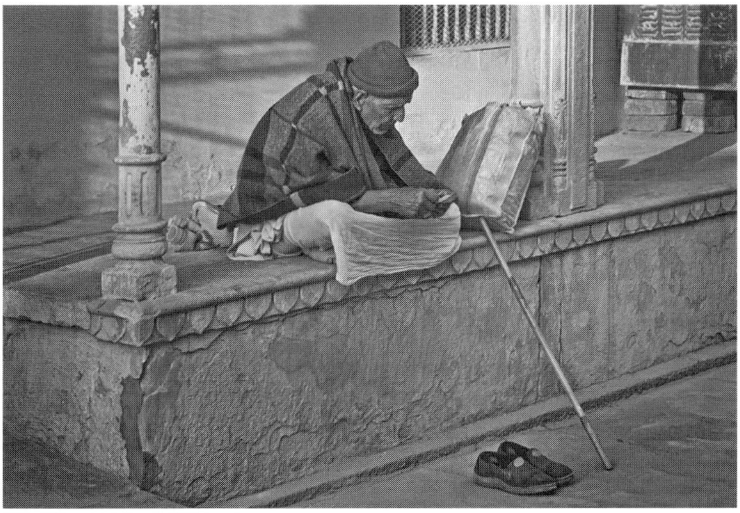

When you're finished, share your ideas with a partner or small group. Add any new ideas you hear.

Listening Activity

Listen to a nurse provide tips to a woman whose father was recently diagnosed with Alzheimer's disease. Write in the missing words in the excerpts below.

1. So, as I mentioned before, your father will experience changes with his __________________ , as well as daily __________________ .
2. We'll provide you with some __________________ that will explain many of those changes and how you and your family can __________________ with them.
3. Try to keep the same __________________ for daily activities, including meals, taking __________________ , bathing, as well as doing hobbies he enjoys.
4. Although there will be __________________ moments for you and your family, it's important to realize that your father may also experience frustration.
5. Above all, be __________________ and __________________ . Tell your father what you are going to do, step by step while you do it.

Speaking Activity

Choose a partner and decide who will play the role of the medical professional and Ms. Akasaka from the listening activity above. Role-play the same situation: Ms. Akasaka's father was diagnosed with Alzheimer's disease, and she will have to take care of him, but needs some guidance from the medical professional. The medical professional will offer the same advice from the listening activity, as well as any new advice you or your partner can think of. Ms. Akasaka will discuss difficulties she may be having, along with questions about the advice. When you are finished, switch roles. You may choose to write out a script first before beginning the role play.

Discussion Questions

1. How are elderly people shown respect in your community? Do you believe that young people are forgetting to respect their elders?
2. Share what you wrote about in the writing section on issues with an aging society. What are some possible solutions for supporting an aging society's physical and mental health?
3. Are you interested in becoming a geriatrician? If not, in what ways do you plan to help elderly people with their medical needs?

Speaking Strategies: Presentation Structure, Part III

Finally, we come to the *conclusion*—the final statement given to an audience to solidify the message of the presentation, speech, or essay. You have laid out your introduction and have explained and supported your main points. The good news is that the hard work is done! All that remains is to summarize your main points, thank your audience, and then check if anyone has any questions. (Note: These final two steps can be omitted if you are writing an essay) . Let's break down these three final steps.

Final Unit Assignment

Topic What Can Medical Students Learn from TV Medical Dramas?

Watch a medical drama (for example, *House, M.D.*) or comedy (for example, *Scrubs*) on television or online, and take notes of any parts that could teach medical students about life as a doctor, nurse, or other medical professional. It could be as simple as the clothing the characters wore ("doctors and nurses wore scrubs") or as complex as the explanation of a surgery to a patient. Write as many points as possible, and either write or present your top three. You can use the chart below to help structure your paper or presentation.

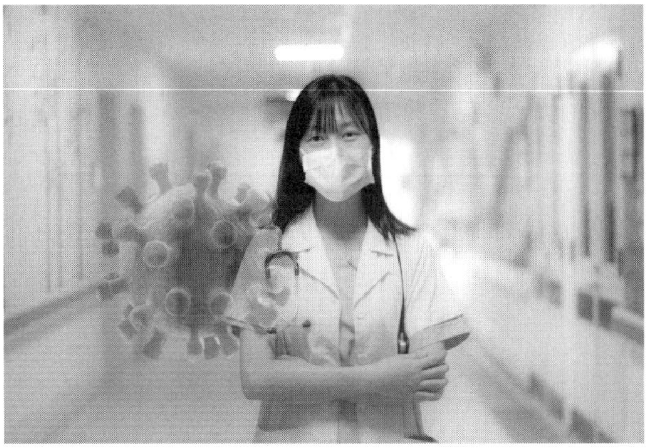

Main Point #	Main Point	Support
1		
2		
3		

UNIT

14 Cultural Considerations

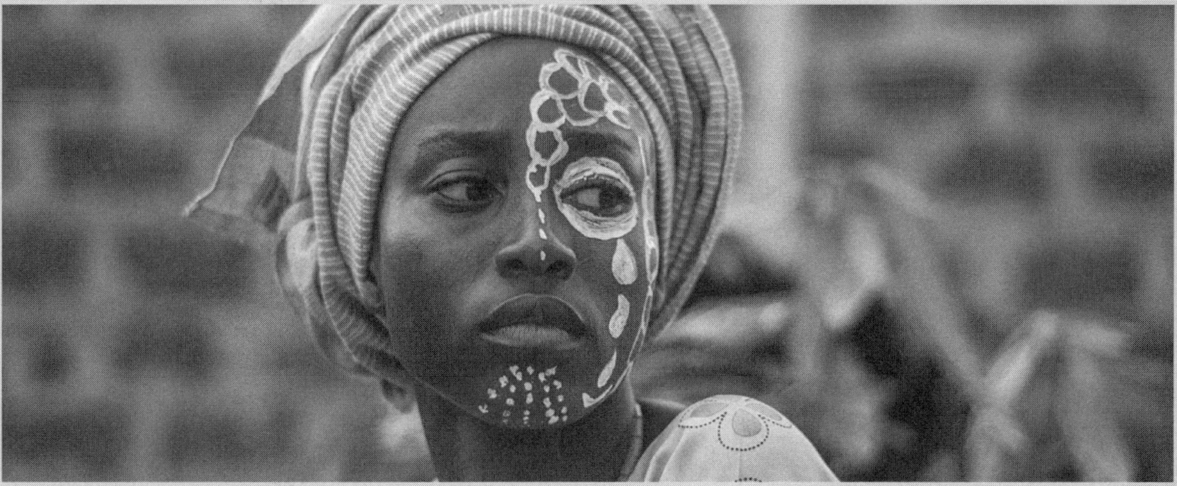

Medical Terms

1. over-the-counter medicine	市販薬 (しはんやく)
2. prescription medicine	処方薬 (しょほうやく)
3. dosage	投薬量 (とうやくりょう)
4. expiration date	使用期限 (しようきげん), 消費期限 (しょうひきげん)
5. liquid medicine	水薬 (みずぐすり)
6. syrup	シロップ
7. powder medicine	粉薬 (こなぐすり)
8. sublingual medicine	舌下錠 (ぜっかじょう)
9. throat lozenge	のど飴 (あめ)
10. capsule	カプセル剤 (ざい)
11. tablet	錠剤 (じょうざい)
12. eye drops	点眼薬 (てんがんやく)
13. ear drops	点耳薬 (てんじやく)
14. ointment	軟膏 (なんこう)
15. suppository	坐薬 (ざやく)
16. enema	浣腸 (かんちょう)
17. anti-inflammatory drug	抗炎症薬 (こうえんしょうやく)
18. antitussive (cough medicine)	鎮咳薬 (ちんがいやく)
19. aspirin	アスピリン
20. ibuprofen	イブプロフェン

21. acetaminophen	アセトアミノフェン
22. painkiller	痛み止め (いたみどめ), 鎮痛剤 (ちんつうざい)
23. sleep medication	睡眠　薬 (すいみんやく)
24. sedative	鎮静剤 (ちんせいざい)
25. diuretic	利尿薬 (りにょうやく)
26. laxative	下剤 (げざい)
27. anti-diarrhea medicine	下痢止め (げりどめ)
28. antibiotic	抗生剤 (こうせいざい), 抗生物質 (こうせいぶっしつ)
29. penicillin	ペニシリン
30. nasal spray	鼻 (はな) づまりスプレー
31. antihistamine	抗 (こう) ヒスタミン剤 (ざい)
32. home remedy	民間療法 (みんかんりょうほう)
33. vitamins	ビタミン
34. Chinese medicine	漢方薬 (かんぽうやく)
35. gargle	うがい
36. swallow	飲み込む (のみこむ)
37. placebo	偽薬 (ぎやく), プラセボ
38. side effects	副作用 (ふくさよう)
39. poison	毒 (どく)
40. antidote	解毒剤 (げどくざい)

Medical Terms: Practice

Look at the pictures below. Write the English name for each one.

1.

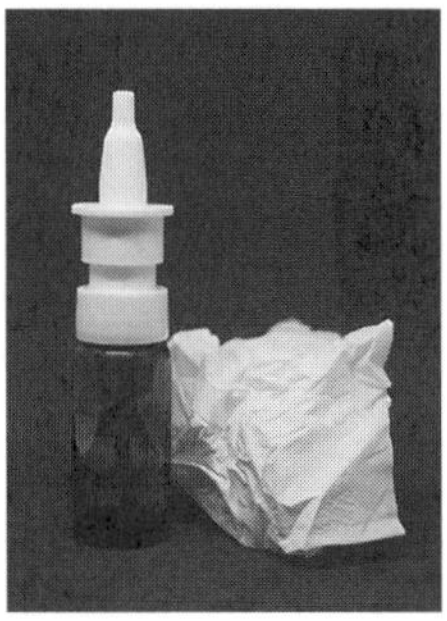

____

2.

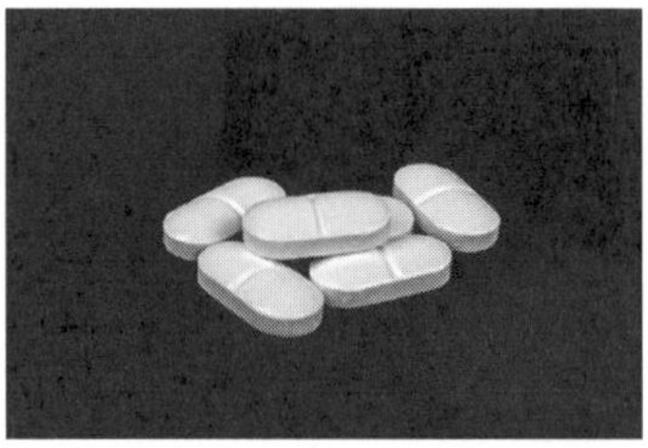

____

3.

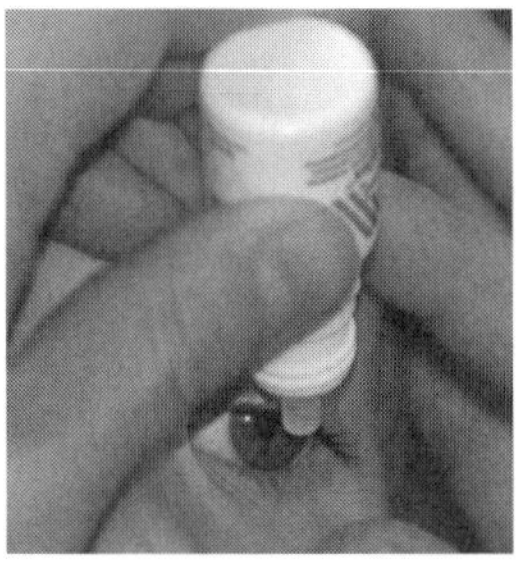

____

4.

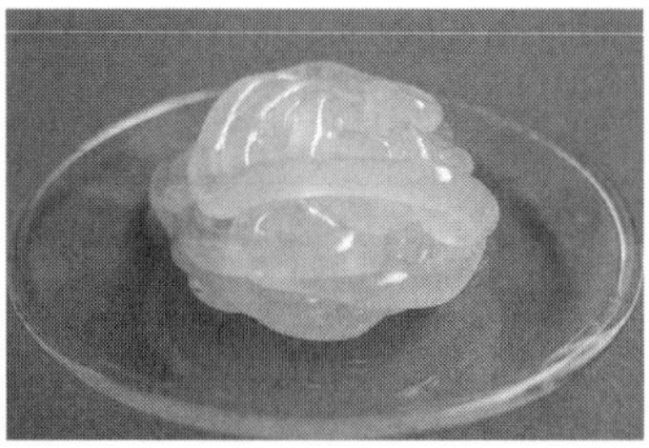

____

5.

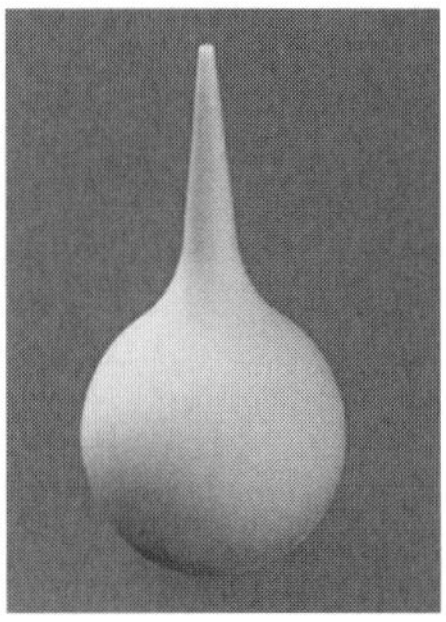

____

6.

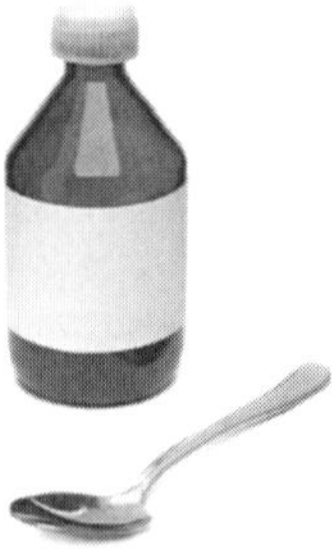

____

7.

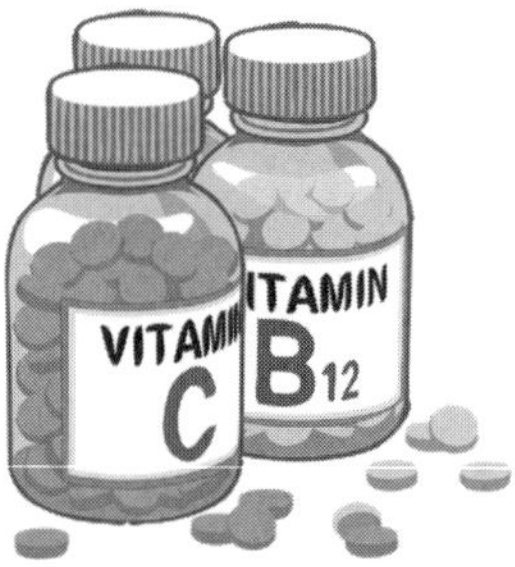

____

8.

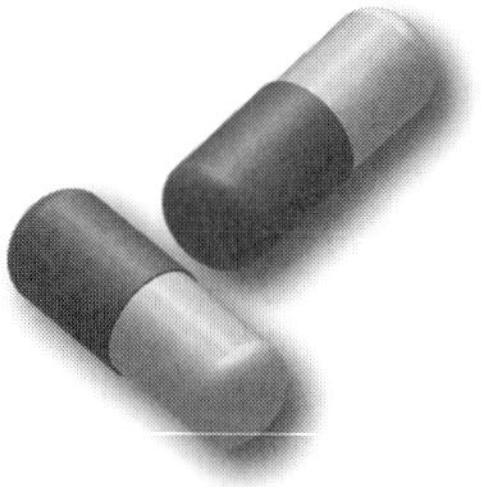

____

Grammar Review: Past Progressive

In the previous unit, you learned about the present progressive, which is also known as the present continuous. In this unit, you will learn about the past progressive, which is also known as the past continuous. Like the present continuous, the past continuous describes an ongoing action or event that happened in the past.

To make the past progressive, use the past form of the verb *be* (was/were) plus a present participle (the -ing form of a verb, or -ing participle) .

The doctor **was** perform*ing* a physical exam.
The nurses **were** discuss*ing* the new patient.

The past progressive can also be written in the negative (wasn't/weren't) , as well as in question form.

The doctor **wasn't** perform*ing* a physical exam.
Weren't the nurses discuss*ing* a new patient?

The past progressive is also used to describe an action or event while a new action or event takes place. We usually use words like *when* and *while* after the past progressive tense to show that the secondary action or event is happening at the same time.

The doctor **was** perform*ing* a physical exam when the phone rang.
The nurses **were** discuss*ing* the new patient while the doctor examined her.

• Grammar Activity 1

Unscramble the words and phrases to make sentences.

1. because / of / wasn't / The / religious / healthy / patient / pork / reasons. / eating

____

2. a / doctor / the / to / child's / mother. / translator / The / was / email / using

____

3. Spain / late / patient / for / Wasn't / appointment? / the / last / her / from

____

4. to / the / next / nurses / were / the/ lunch / halal / restaurant / eating / The / at / clinic.

____

5. patient's / the / called / The / checking / nurse / doctors / her. / when / the / were / chart

____

• Grammar Activity 2

Complete the dialogue with the correct verb tense.

Student A: What ____________ you ___________ (do) last night?

Student B: I ______________ ________________ (watch) YouTube. Why?

Student A: I ______________ ________________ (try) to call you!

Student B: ______________you ________________ (call) me? I didn't ________________ (receive) any calls.

Student A: ______________you ________________ (cancel) the calls?

Student B: Why would I ______________ (do) that?

Student A: What ______________ you ________________ (watch) on YouTube?

Student B: I ______________ ________________ (watch) last week's online lesson on cultural misunderstandings in medicine ... and some cute cat videos.

Student A: I knew it! That's why you ______________ ______________ (ignore) my calls.

Student B: Sorry.

• Grammar Activity 3

Complete the questions with the past progressive.

1. What ______________ ______________(happen) at the hospital during the earthquake?

2. During the pandemic, the governmen ______________ ______________(promote) the new vaccine developed in the U.S.

3. The hospital ______________ ______________ (decide) how to increase satisfaction rates among foreign patients.

4. This time last year, the number of foreign nurses working in Japan ______________

_______________ (increase) by 20%.

5. The hiring committee _______________ _______________ (consider) two Sri Lankan candidates for the hospital residency.

Reading with Fushigi-chan: Culture and Medicine

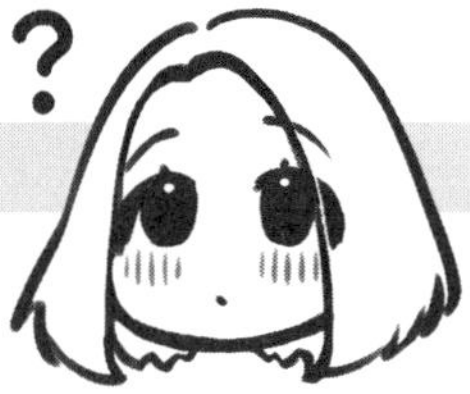

As more people move to new countries to live and work, the need for medical attention will increase. These interactions may lead to cultural misunderstandings, which is when one culture misunderstands another culture's actions, beliefs, or words. This can be an extremely frustrating, embarrassing, and sometimes even dangerous situation depending on the country and context. Cultural misunderstandings that happen during a vacation are one thing, but imagine how much more critical it can be in a medical situation.

Before we can discuss some cultural differences and misunderstandings that could happen in medical settings, it is important to understand the term *ethnocentrism* (民族中心主義, みんぞくちゅうしんしゅぎ). Ethnocentrism happens when one culture judges another culture based on their own cultural beliefs. It's a natural occurrence, but the big problem with ethnocentrism is thinking "my culture is better than yours." In medicine, it is very important that doctors, nurses and other medical professionals have an open mind to cultural differences and beliefs, especially when those differences and beliefs involve healing practices.

Not every culture views healing in the same way. While most Westernized societies have hospitals with highly trained staff, high-tech medical equipment, and modern medicines that handle a variety of illnesses and diseases, some cultures believe that illness and disease come from divine punishment, bad luck, spirits, or other supernatural forces (Murdock, et al., 1978).

Treatment for certain ailments will also vary and will differ greatly from a Westernized approach to healing. In Canada, for example, an ill person would be examined by a doctor or nurse, given certain tests (blood test, x-ray, etc.), and often prescribed medication that has undergone extensive testing before being offered to the public. In Uganda, however, a person may be "prescribed massage, sweat baths, cupping with a horn, blistering with a hot iron, or the internal or external use of various herbal remedies" (Murdock, et al., 1978, p. 449). While this may sound strange or even unethical to some people, it is important to understand and accept that there is no "best" way, but instead many different ways to treat illness based on cultural beliefs and practices.

Another aspect of culture that must be considered when providing medical treatment is religion. Depending on the religious belief, there may be certain medical restrictions that doctors and other medical professionals must be aware of and respect. Jehovah's Witnesses, for example, do not accept blood transfusions and will refuse to have an autopsy done on a corpse unless it is required by law (Metropolitan Chicago Healthcare Council, n.d.) . These restrictions are based on their understanding and interpretation of the Bible and must be respected by physicians and other medical professionals.

This can be easier said than done. In 2015, a 14-year-old leukemia patient died after refusing a blood transfusion that would have given him a 70% chance of surviving the next five years (Fox News, 2015) . In another case, a 15-year-old boy also died after refusing a blood transfusion based on his religious beliefs (Guardian, 2010) .

The examples from Uganda and Jehovah's Witnesses are not intended to paint them in a negative light, but to illustrate how cultural differences and beliefs may interact with medical practices. The goal as medical professionals is to provide quality medical care to patients while respecting their culture, gender, and other characteristics and qualities that make them unique individuals.

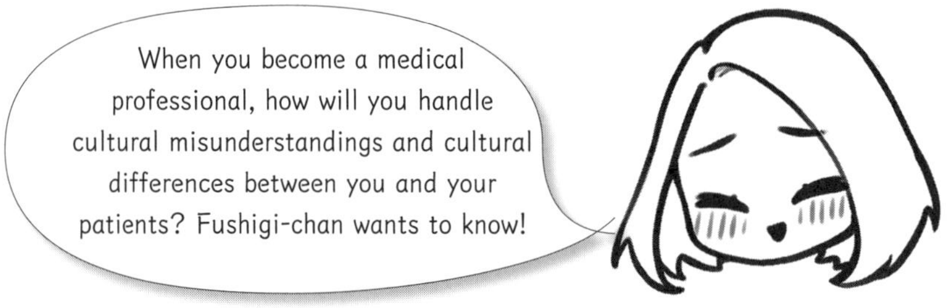

• Reading Activity 1

Circle (T) if the statement is true or (F) if the statement is false.

1. Cultural misunderstandings only happen when you travel abroad. (T・F)
2. Jehovah's Witnesses prescribe sweat baths to ill people. (T・F)
3. Non-Western approaches to medicine are unethical. (T・F)
4. Different cultures view healing in different ways. (T・F)
5. Some cultures believe supernatural forces cause sickness. (T・F)

• Reading Activity 2

Fill in the blanks with the appropriate words.

1. The belief that one culture is superior to another culture is called ______________ .

2. Some religions don't allow believers to receive blood ______________ or have ______________ conducted on them when they die.

3. It's important for medical professionals to have an ______________ ______________ to cultural differences and beliefs.

4. If the 14-year-old leukemia patient received a blood transfusion, he would have had a ______________ chance of surviving the next ______________ years.

5. Some cultures believe that sickness come from divine ______________ , bad ______________ , spirits, or other ______________ forces.

Writing Activity

Have you ever experienced a cultural misunderstanding? Write 4 or 5 sentences describing your experience in the box below. If you have never experienced a cultural misunderstanding, think about an experience you heard about from a family member or friend, or a situation in a television show or movie.

When you're finished, share your writing with a partner or the class.

Listening Activity

Listen to a woman talk about cultural differences she encountered when visiting a doctor in a foreign country. What was her health problem? What was she surprised by? What medical care did she receive, and what were the cultural differences she experienced? While you listen, write your notes below. Afterwards, discuss them with your partner or small group.

Speaker's name:________________

Health issue:____

Surprised by:____

Medical care received: ____

Cultural differences:____

Speaking Activity

Without looking at what you wrote in the Writing Activity, describe your cultural misunderstanding story. When did it happen? Where were you? Who was involved? What was the situation? How was it solved?

When you finish, listen to your partner's story. Take notes below.

Partner's name: ________________

His/her story:

____

____

____

____

____

____

____

Now find a new partner and tell him or her your previous partner's story.

Discussion Questions

1. Some countries that are mainly monocultural (the majority of the population is the same culture or ethnicity) often have a difficult time accepting those who are different from them. However, with issues such as declining birthrates and aging societies, they are left with little choice but to accept more foreigners into their countries. What are some ways hospitals can better prepare for foreigners who require medical attention?
2. What are some common stereotypes (mostly false and often negative beliefs about a group of people) in your community about people from other groups? Can you think of ways these stereotypical beliefs are connected to health care?
3. In this reading section, examples were used to show how different cultures can be from one another. Think of a story, movie, television show, news report, etc., that illustrates cultural differences and/or different cultures coming to understand and accept each other. Share the story with a partner or small group.

Speaking Strategies: The Outline and Preparation

Every good speech, presentation or essay needs a plan, and this section will cover the basics of a good outline, as well as preparation tips for any upcoming speaking project. There are many outline formats available in books and online resources, so it is recommended to find one that suits your style of research and speaking. You can also combine the **Speaking Strategies** sections from the last two units to make a complete outline for a presentation or speech.

Final Unit Assignment

Topic Non-Verbal Communication

Non-verbal communication is the way people communicate using their body. This includes facial expressions, gestures, and posture. Think about the ways people in your country use non-verbal communication. Research another country's non-verbal communication, and then compare the similarities and differences.

After you have collected enough material to support your ideas, it's time to create an outline. Although you may use the format of your choice to create an outline for your presentation, your instructor can also provide the Outline Form based on the previous units. You may also use the Venn diagram below. When you have finished, share your outline with a partner and your instructor, and write down any feedback you receive.

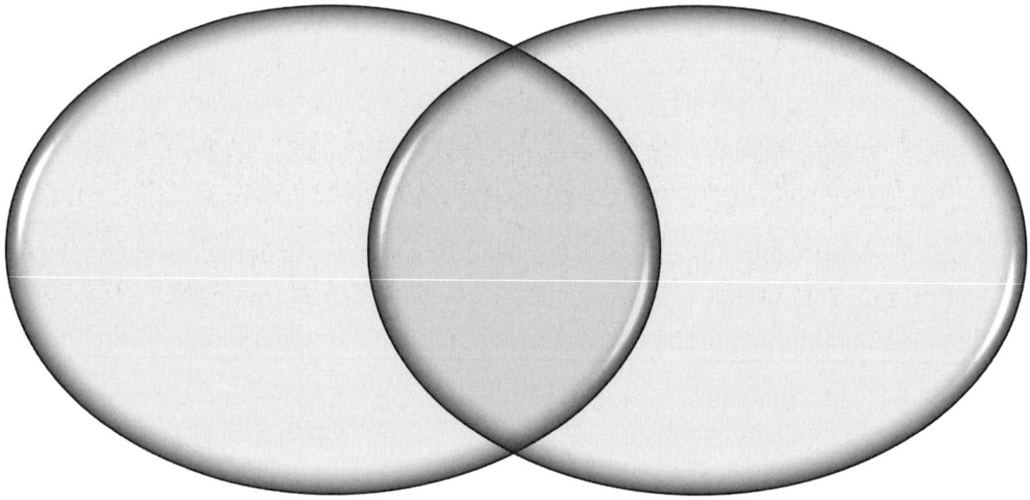

UNIT 15

End of Life Care

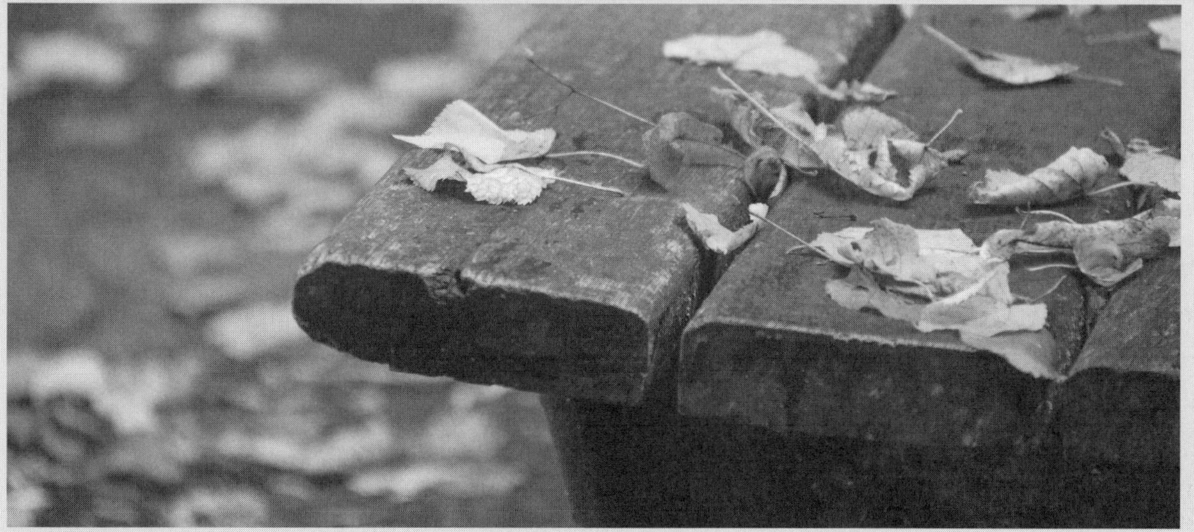

Medical Terms

1. medical university	医科大学 (いかだいがく)
2. school of medicine	医学科 (いがくか)
3. national examination for doctors	医師国家試験 (いしこっかしけん)
4. Doctor of Medicine (M.D.)	医学博士 (いがくはくし)
5. school of nursing	看護学科 (かんごがっか)
6. clinical nursing	臨床看護学 (りんしょうかんごがく)
7. maternity nursing	母性看護学 (ぼせいかんごがく)
8. scrubs	医療用 (いりょうよう) スクラブ
9. lab coat	白衣 (はくい)
10. rounds	回診 (かいしん)
11. autopsy	検死解剖 (けんしかいぼう)
12. cadaver	[解剖用] 死体 ([かいぼうよう] したい)
13. anatomy	解剖学 (かいぼうがく)
14. human dissection	人体解剖 (じんたいかいぼう)
15. medical ethics	医療倫理 (いりょうりんり)
16. physiology	生理学 (せいりがく)
17. microbiology	微生物学 (びせいぶつがく)
18. physics	物理学 (ぶつりがく)
19. chemistry	化学 (かがく)
20. solvent	溶媒 (ようばい)

21. biology	生物学 (せいぶつがく)
22. oxygen	酸素 (さんそ)
23. carbon dioxide	炭酸 (たんさん) ガス, 二酸化炭素 (にさんかたんそ)
24. osteology	骨学 (こつがく)
25. genetics	遺伝学 (いでんがく)
26. deoxyribonucleic acid (DNA)	デオキシリボ核酸 (かくさん)
27. gene	遺伝子 (いでんし)
28. heredity	遺伝 (いでん)
29. epidemiology	疫学 (えきがく)
30. mutation	突然変異 (とつぜんへんい)
31. organism	生命体 (せいめいたい)
32. immunology	免疫学 (めんえきがく)
33. hemoglobin	ヘモグロビン
34. enzyme	酵素 (こうそ)
35. sucrose	スクロース
36. in vivo	生体内 (せいたいない)
37. sedimentation	沈殿 (ちんでん)
38. pharmacology	薬理学 (やくりがく)
39. statistics	統計学 (とうけいがく)
40. mathematics	数学 (すうがく)

Medical Terms: Practice

Match the medical terms (1-10) to their definitions (a-j).

1) ____ autopsy •	• a. the study of bones
2) ____ epidemiology •	• b. branch of medicine dealing with the uses and effects of drugs
3) ____ enzyme •	• c. a dead body
4) ____ heredity •	• d. substance produced by living organisms that helps with chemical reactions
5) ____ immunology •	• e. branch of medicine that deals with occurrence and control of a disease
6) ____ osteology •	• f. characteristics passed on from parent to child
7) ____ genetics •	• g. branch of medicine dealing with immunity
8) ____ in vivo •	• h. examination of a dead body to determine the cause of death
9) ____ cadaver •	• i. taking place inside a living organism
10) ____ pharmacology •	• j. the study of genes and heredity

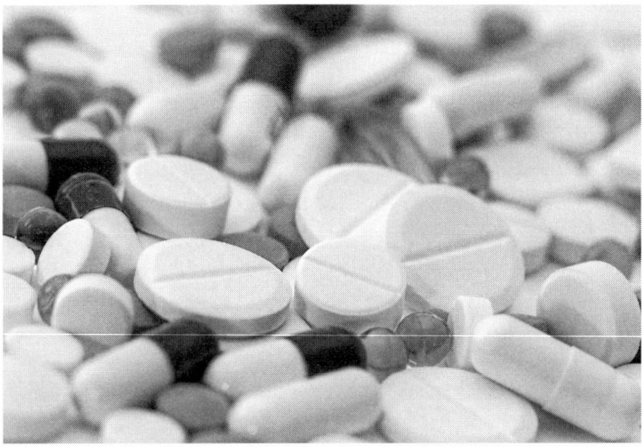

Grammar Review: Past Progressive

The final grammar review will focus on the future. Most of you probably already know that the future is made by using the verb *be + going to* or *will + the base form of a verb*. However, many students don't really understand the correct ways to use each one.

We use *be + going to* to talk about plans for the future, and when you are certain something is going to happen.

Kaho **is** *going to* apply for an internship in Australia.
She was accepted? I'**m** *going to* miss her so much!

We use *will + the base form of a verb* to talk about our predictions or factual events in the future.

The number of nurses in Japan **will decrease** next year.
Next year's international exposition **will be** held in Osaka.

Here is a general rule to follow: Use *going to* when having informal conversations and discussing plans and intentions for the future. Use *will* for predictions, expectations, and factual events in the future.

After I become a doctor, I'**m going to** buy a house.
After I become a doctor, I **will buy** a house.

While the second sentence isn't incorrect, it is better to use *going to* because this is a plan for the future (and it seems like this would be a casual conversation) .

The new hospital **will not be** ready until 2025.
The new hospital **is not going to** be ready until 2025.

Again, the second sentence isn't incorrect, but since this is a prediction/expectation for the future (and it seems like an official statement) , it is best to use *will*.

Here are three more ways to talk about the future.

1) You can also use *may / might + the base form of a verb* to talk about the future.

Kaho **may** *stay* in Australia after her internship.
She **might** *present* at the next medical conference in Tokyo.

2) You can use the **present progressive** (see **Unit 13**) to talk about plans for the future that were usually decided beforehand.

Kaho **is** apply*ing* for an internship in Australia.
When **are** you graduat*ing* from medical school?

3) You can use *will* to talk about decisions that are made at the moment you are speaking.

"We need a surgeon in ER now!" "I'**ll do** it."
Will you **help** me with this lab report?

• Grammar Activity 1

Complete the phone conversation between a patient and clinic staff. Circle *be going to* or *will*. If both choices are possible, circle both answers.

Staff: Omiya Health Clinic. How can I help you?

Patient: Hello. This is Haruka Morita. I requested a home visit for this morning, but a doctor hasn't arrived. (**Are you going to** / **Will you**) send a doctor soon?

Staff: Hello Haruka. Yes, I (**am going to** / **will**) .

Patient: (**Will they** / **Are they going to**) arrive soon? My condition is getting worse.

Staff: I'm very sorry. The clinic has been unusually busy today. Dr. Suda (**will** / **is going to**) leave the clinic in 10 minutes.

Patient: (**Are you going to** / **Will you**) send Dr. Williams instead? He is already familiar with my condition.

Staff: I understand. I (**will** / **am going to**) see if Dr. Williams is available.

Patient: Thank you very much. I appreciate it.

• Grammar Activity 2

Use the time expressions in the box below to make questions. Write your questions below. When you're finished, ask a partner the questions to find out about their plans for the near future.

this weekend	tomorrow	at 18:00	tonight	next year

1.____

2.____

3. ____

4. ____

5. ____

• Grammar Activity 3

Use *will* + the verb in parentheses to talk about the future of medicine.

1. Every elderly person ________________ (have) a robotic nurse.
2. Future hospitals ________________ (run) on solar and wind energy.
3. Hospital cafeterias ________________ (grow) their own vegetables on the roof.
4. Patients ________________ (not pay) for prescription medication.
5. Medical students ________________ (get) all their textbooks for free!

Reading with Fushigi-chan: Life and Death

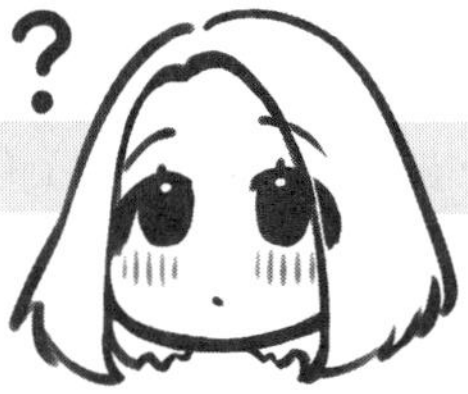

Being a doctor, nurse, or other professional in the medical field can be an extremely rewarding job filled with many wonderful and amazing moments. From delivering a woman's first baby to helping a patient overcome a serious disease, doctors, nurses, and other members of a medical team can be a part of happy memories that a patient will remember forever. Unfortunately, although everyone starts out as babies taking their first breath, we will also, sadly, one day take our last breath. When a person is nearing death—the last stage of a human being's life cycle—it is important for medical professionals to understand and provide, as best as possible, what a patient needs at the end of his or her life.

End-of-life care is the care that is provided to patients when they are very close to dying. Depending on the situation, a patients can be hours, days, or even months away from dying, so one of the first decisions that needs to be made is where the patient wishes to spend the remainder of their time. Some patients choose to stay at home while others choose to remain in a hospital. For people who are terminally ill, there are special places called *hospices* （ホスピス） that provide end-of-life care.

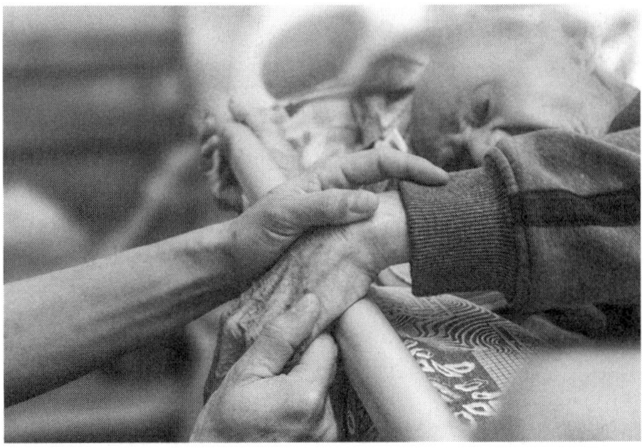

Regardless of where the patient is, it is critical that patients who are dying are as comfortable as possible. If a medical professional is providing end-of-life care, they must make sure to address any pain the patient is experiencing, problems breathing, and any other issues, such as digestive issues or skin irritations. Relieving these symptoms without trying to cure the causes is called *palliative treatment* and is a very important part of end-of-life care.

Doctors, nurses, and other medical staff are there to ensure the patient is as comfortable as possible, but sometimes uncomfortable feelings don't come from a physical source, but a mental one. Patients who are close to dying can experience a variety of feelings, including sadness or depression, anxiety, and even anger. Medical professionals are there to tend to their medical needs, but if the patient needs additional support, there are still things that can be done to help. One of the first acts that should be taken is to contact the in-hospital counselor who is trained to provide mental health support. If one is not available, a recommendation can be made to the family to seek out this type of care.

There are other areas involved in end-of-life care, including final wishes, requests to take care of a home or pet, and perhaps even spiritual needs. It is not part of a medical professional's duties to become involved in these matters, but some patients or their family members may ask medical staff about these matters, so they must be prepared to refer them to relevant individuals, businesses and organizations that may be able to help.

Caring for a patient who is at the end of their life can be physically, mentally, and emotionally challenging. Being prepared, showing empathy and compassion, and providing the best medical care that is possible are ways to help patients and families cope with this final stage in life.

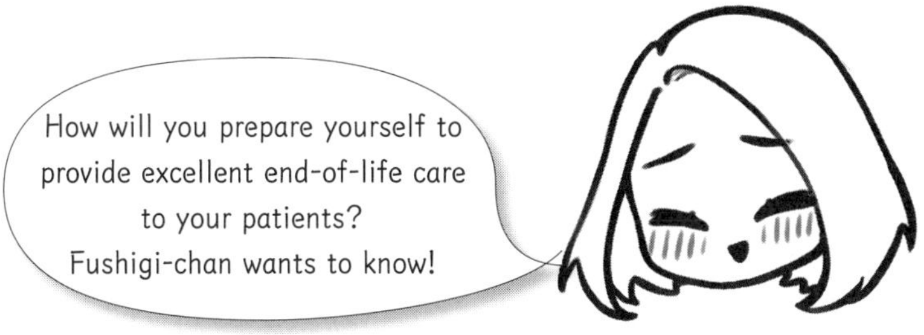

• Reading Activity 1

Circle (T) if the statement is true or (F) if the statement is false.

1. End-of-life care includes physical, mental, and emotional needs. (T・F)

2. Doctors and nurses should provide mental health support. (T・F)

3. When patients are dying, they sometimes have digestive issues. (T・F)

4. A hospice is the same as a hospital. (T・F)

5. Patients expect doctors and nurses to care for them spiritually. (T・F)

• Reading Activity 2

Fill in the blanks with the appropriate words.

1. Relieving a patient's symptoms without trying to cure the cause is called ________________ .

2. If a patient is experiencing depression or anxiety, contact a person who is trained to provide ______________ ______________ ______________ .

3. Other areas involved in end-of-life care include ______________ wishes and ______________ needs.

4. If you are providing end-of-life care, make sure you address any ______________ the patient is experiencing, problems ______________ , and ______________ issues or ______________ irritations.

5. Caring for a patient who is at the end of their life can be both ______________ and ______________ draining.

Writing Activity

Imagine that, as a patient, you are nearing the end of your life. What are some final wishes and requests that you would have? Write 4 or 5 wishes and requests in the box below. After you finish writing, think about how you would respond to these wishes and requests as a doctor, nurse, or other medical professional. Write 2 or 3 sentences about how you would respond to your patient and what you would do for him or her.

When you're finished, share your writing with a partner or the class.

Listening Activity

Listen to a nurse talk about providing end-of-life care for patients. After you finish listening, answer the questions below.

1. What is the nurse's name and age, and how long has she been a nurse?

2. Where does she currently work as a nurse?

3. What is the meaning that the nurse gives for end-of-life care?

____

____

4. What are two pieces of advice that the nurse gives to new doctors and nurses?

____

____

5. What is the final point the nurse makes about providing end-of-life care?

____

____

Speaking Activity

Bronnie Ware is an Australian palliative caregiver who cared for people on their deathbed. While caring for them, she learned about their lives and the regrets they had. She collected their stories and put together the five most common regrets people who were about to die had about their lives. They are:

1. "I wish I'd had the courage to live a life true to myself, not the life others expected of me."
2. "I wish I hadn't worked so hard."
3. "I wish I'd had the courage to express my feelings."
4. "I wish I had stayed in touch with my friends."
5. "I wish that I had let myself be happier." (Ware, 2012)

What are your thoughts on the top five regrets people have? Which ones are you afraid you might have later in life? Explain your reasons to your partner. What other regrets do you think you might have?

When you finish, listen to your partner, and take notes on what he or she said.

Lastly, offer some advice to each other on ways you both can change your lives to remove one or more regrets from your lists.

Partner's name: ____________________

His/her regrets:

1. ____

2. ____

3. ____

4. ____

5. ____

Discussion Questions

1. What do you think will be the most difficult part of providing end-of-life care to patients? What ways can it become less difficult?

2. Do you believe there is enough support for caregivers—family members and professional caregivers who are in charge of providing some or all of the care for terminally ill patients? What can be done to provide more support?

3. Why do you think final wishes, last requests, and spiritual guidance become important for patients who are reaching the end of their lives? Should medical professionals become involved in these areas or are they best left to family members?

Speaking Strategies: Review

Consider all the speaking strategies that were presented in this textbook. Review each unit and write brief summaries or "highlights" of each point. What were the important takeaways?

Final Unit Assignment

Topic Topics in End-of-Life Care

Choose a topic related to end-of-life care. For example, *handling anxiety and depression in patients who are nearing the end of life* or *addressing the needs of caregivers for terminally ill patients*.

After you choose a topic, conduct research, and write an outline for a presentation or paper. You can use the outline form in this textbook or create your own.

Using your outline and research notes, give a presentation or write your paper. Alternatively, you can simply discuss your research in a casual yet organized small-group discussion.

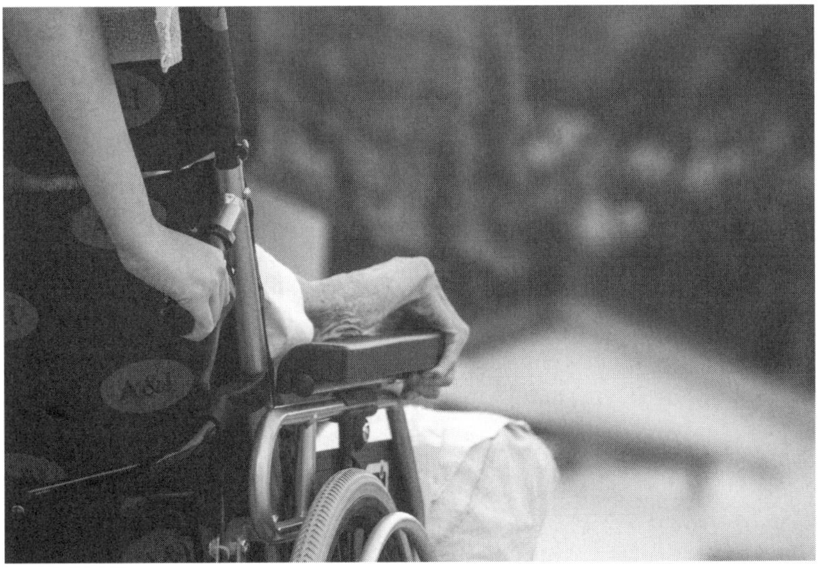

References

Baile, W. F., Buckman, R., Lenzi, R., Glober, G., Beale, E. A., & Kudelka, A. P. (2000) . SPIKES-A six-step protocol for delivering bad news: application to the patient with cancer. The oncologist, 5 (4) , 302–311.https://doi.org/10.1634/theoncologist.5-4- 302

Centers for Disease Control and Prevention (2022) . CDC's Developmental Milestones. Retrieved from https://www.cdc.gov/ncbddd/actearly/milestones/index.html

Center for Disease Control and Prevention. (2022) . Obesity and Overweight. Retrieved from https://www.cdc.gov/nchs/fastats/obesity-overweight.htm

Ferlay, J., Ervik, M., Lam, F, Colombet, M., Mery, L., Piñeros, M., et al. (2020) . Global Cancer Observatory: Cancer Today. Lyon: International Agency for Research on Cancer.

Fox News. (2015) . Teen Jehovah's Witness Leukemia Patient Dies After Refusing Blood Transfusion. Retrieved from https://www.foxnews.com/story/teen-jehovahs-witness-leukemia-patient-dies-after-refusing-blood-transfusion

Guardian. (2010) . Jehovah's Witness teenager dies after refusing blood transfusion. Retrieved from https://www.theguardian.com/uk/2010/may/18/jehovahs-witness-dies-refuse-blood-transfusion

Guinness World Records. (2021) . Most children delivered at a single birth to survive. Retrieved from https://www.guinnessworldrecords.com/world-records/most-children-delivered-at-a-single-birth-to-survive

Guinness World Records. (2022) . Oldest person to give birth. Retrieved from https://www.guinnessworldrecords.com/world-records/oldest-person-to-give-birth

Harvey, A. M. (1973) . Our medical heritage: some examples of creative scholarship. Phar Alpha Omega Alpha.

Kooij, I. A., Sahami, S., Meijer, S. L., Buskens, C. J., & Te Velde, A. A. (2016) . The immunology of the vermiform appendix: a review of the literature. Clinical and experimental immunology, 186 (1) , 1–9. https://doi.org/10.1111/cei.12821

Labella, A. M., Merel, S. E., & Phelan, E. A. (2011) . Ten ways to improve the care of elderly patients in the hospital. Journal of hospital medicine, 6 (6) , 351–357. https://doi.org/10.1002/jhm.900

Metropolitan Chicago Healthcare Council. (n.d.) . Guidelines for Health Care Providers Interacting With Jehovah's Witnesses and Their Families. Retrieved from https://www.advocatehealth.com › assets › documents › faith › cgjehovahs_witnesses.pdf

Murdock, G. P., Wilson, S. F., & Frederick, V. (1978) . World Distribution of Theories of Illness. Ethnology, 17 (4) , 449–470. https://doi.org/10.2307/3773194

Nahin, R. L., Dahlhamer, J. M., & Stussman, B. J. (2010) . Health need and the use of alternative medicine among adults who do not use conventional medicine. BMC health services research, 10, 220. https://doi.org/10.1186/1472-6963-10-220

National Cancer Institute. (2022) . Common Cancer Types. Retrieved from https://www.cancer.gov/types/common-cancers

National Center for Chronic Disease Prevention and Health Promotion. (2022) . Promoting Health for Adults. Retrieved from https://www.cdc.gov/chronicdisease/resources/publications/factsheets/promoting-health-for-adults.htm

Time. (1945) . Medicine: Prodigious Pregnancy. Retrieved from https://content.time.com/time/subscriber/article/0,33009,797153,00.html

U.S. Department of Health and Human Services. (2022) . Alzheimers.gov: Tips for caregivers and families of people with Dementia. Retrieved from https://www.alzheimers.gov/life-with-dementia/tips-caregivers

USA Today. (2017) . Mom pleads with doctor to resuscitate baby delivered at 21 weeks. Retrieved from https://www.usatoday.com/story/news/nation-now/2017/11/14/mom-delivers-earliest-premature-baby-ever-and-chooses-resuscitate-miracle-aughter-now-healthy-toddle/861386001/

World Health Organization. (2017) . Mental health of older adults. Retrievedfrom https://www.who.int/en/news-room/fact-sheets/detail/mental-health-of-older-adults

World Health Organization. (2020) . Cancer. Retrieved from https://www.who.int/news-room/fact-sheets/detail/cancer

World Health Organization. (2022) . Age-friendly World. Retrieved from https://extranet.who.int/agefriendlyworld/afp/

World Health Organization. (2022) . Obesity and overweight. Retrieved from https://www.who.int/news-room/fact-sheets/detail/obesity-and-overweight

World Obesity. (2022) . Global Obesity Observation. Retrieved from https://data.worldobesity.org/rankings/?age=c&sex=m

Photographs and Images

All photographs and images are taken from https://pixabay.com or https://unsplash.com/. Photographs and images from Pixabay and Unspalsh are free to use for commercial use with no attribution required.

Disclaimer

Any website mentioned in this textbook, either in-text or in the reference list, is neither endorsed by nor connected to the author or the publisher. At the time of publication, all websites listed in this textbook were checked by the author to ensure they provided the information that they claim to give. However, information on websites rapidly changes, and so the author and the publishers cannot and will not be held legally responsible for any of the content found on any website that is used while completing activities in this textbook.

About the Author

Dr. Daniel Velasco is a university professor and mental health therapist in Japan.

Acknowledgements

I would like to thank the following individuals for their contributions to this textbook.

Review Team

-Dr. Gregory Glasgow: Dr. Glasgow is an Associate Professor at Kanda University of International Studies. His latest book is entitled "Multiculturalism, Language, and Race in English Education in Japan: Agency, Pedagogy, and Reckoning". He is interested in how concepts from social theory can be applied to the study of sociolinguistics in language education. He researches language policy, structure/agency, and raciolinguistics in Global Englishes Language Teaching and second language teacher education.

-Dr. Donald Patterson: Dr. Patterson holds an EdD and is a professor in the School of International Education at Seirei Christopher University in Hamamatsu, Japan. He teaches general English courses and ESP courses for students in nursing, rehabilitation, social work, and child education. His research interests include learner mindsets, effort regulation, motivation, and the internationalization of education.

-Dr. Makiko Hayasaka: Dr. Hayasaka obtained degrees in music at the International Christian University and Tokyo University of the Arts, and earned her PhD in musicology at the University of Bristol. She is interested in CLIL and ESP, and is currently developing an English language teaching program for music students. She is currently an Associate Professor at Tokyo College of Music.

-Liz Williams: Ms. Williams is a Tokyo-based JP/ENG translator. For translation inquiries, write to her at lizwilliams.translation@gmail.com.

Artwork

Thank you to Kopa-chan (こぱちゃん) for bringing Fushigi-chan to life. For more information, visit the artist's online portfolio: https://fori.io/chululalila.

Audio and Video

Lastly, a huge thank you to the medical and nursing students at Kindai University (Grace and Hana), Showa University (Minami and Marino), and Seirei Christopher University (Ayaka Hashimoto), as well as other medical students and faculty members who gave their time to record authentic recordings for this textbook. Also, thank you to the professional doctors and nurses who agreed to be interviewed for the recordings. Finally, thank you to the other individuals who shared their experiences as patients.

著者略歴

ダニエル・ヴェラスコ（Daniel Velasco）

2005 年　カリフォルニア大学ロサンジェルス校卒業
2007 年　ナショナル大学大学院修士課程
2009 年　アンティオック大学大学院修士課程
2012 年　シカゴ・スクール・オブ・プロフェッショナル・サイコロジー
　　　　　博士課程修了
2020 年　日本心理学会認定心理士
現　在　近畿大学医学部専任講師
　　　　　博士（心理学）

コミュニケーションのための医学英語
Medical English for Communication　　　定価はカバーに表示

2024 年 3 月 1 日　初版第 1 刷

著　者　ダニエル・ヴェラスコ
発行者　朝　倉　誠　造
発行所　株式会社　朝　倉　書　店
東京都新宿区新小川町 6-29
郵 便 番 号　162-8707
電　話　03（3260）0141
F A X　03（3260）0180
https://www.asakura.co.jp

〈検印省略〉

シナノ印刷・渡辺製本

ISBN 978-4-254-30128-1　C 3047　　　Printed in Japan